The NATURAL HEALING COMPANION

THE
NATURAL
HEALING
COMPANION

USING ALTERNATIVE MEDICINES
WHAT TO BUY, HOW TO TAKE,
AND WHEN TO COMBINE
FOR BEST RESULTS

Dr. Deborah A. Wiancek

NATUROPATHIC PHYSICIAN, CLINICIAN, AND AUTHOR OF
THE COMPLETE NATURAL MEDICINE REFERENCE

RODALE

Printed in the United States of America on acid-free ∞ , recycled paper ♻

Cover Designer: Richard Kershner
Cover and Interior Photographer: Kurt Wilson

Library of Congress Cataloging-in-Publication Data

Wiancek, Deborah A.
    The natural healing companion : using alternative medicines : what to buy, how to take, and when to combine for best results / Deborah A. Wiancek.
        p.   cm.
    Includes index.
    ISBN: 1-57954-245-X   paperback
    1. Naturopathy   2. Alternative medicine.   I. Title.
RZ440.W53   2000
615.5—dc21   00-009348

Distributed to the book trade by St. Martin's Press

2 4 6 8 10 9 7 5 3 1   paperback

Visit us on the Web at www.rodalebooks.com, or call us toll-free at (800) 848-4735.

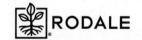

WE **INSPIRE** AND **ENABLE** PEOPLE TO IMPROVE
THEIR LIVES AND THE WORLD AROUND THEM

You probably know someone who gets sick a lot. They catch every cold that comes along, suffer from frequent stomachaches, or complain about chronic sinusitis. And they always seem to get sick at the worst possible time—when they're facing a deadline at work, expecting out-of-town guests, even when they're going on vacation.

People who are frequently ill or who become ill during times of stress often have compromised immune systems. Your immune system is your body's defense against infection, and it is one of the most complex and fascinating systems in the human body. But lifestyle factors—including stress, poor diet, lack of exercise, smoking, and excessive alcohol consumption—can undermine your immune system and cause you to fall ill.

EAT RIGHT TO STAY HEALTHY

The way to stay healthy is to keep your immune system strong, and proper nutrition is the number one way to keep it in good working order. Food is the best medicine of all, provided you eat the right balance of nutrients, proteins, fats, and carbohydrates. Study after study links dietary deficiency to disease.

What constitutes a healthy diet? Specific requirements vary from one person to another, but the following general guidelines will get you off to a good start.

Eat at least five servings of fruits and five servings of vegetables a day. The best way to do this is to eat a salad with five different vegetables in it—the more colorful the salad, the greater the variety of nutrients you are getting. For fruits, eat a fruit salad or several fruit snacks during the day, or sprinkle a variety of fruits on your morning cereal.

Eating fruits and vegetables increases the amount of fiber in your diet and helps you get your required daily quota of vitamins and minerals. The benefits include a reduced risk of disease, lower cholesterol and blood pressure, and help in losing weight. More than 200 studies have shown that eating fruits and vegetables helps protect you from various forms of cancer. Other studies indicate similar protection against cardiovascular disease, diabetes, stroke, diverticulosis, and cataracts.

One piece of fruit or ½ cup of a vegetable constitutes a single serving. Because cooking destroys valuable nutrients, try to eat fruits and vegetables raw, or steam vegetables lightly before eating. Precooked, frozen, and canned fruits and vegetables are lower in nutrients and higher in sodium, sugar, and preservatives.

Eat five servings of whole grains a day. Avoid white bread, white rice, and other heavily processed grains. Even if they are "enriched" or "fortified," they are still lacking essential nutrients. Instead, look for foods made from 100 percent whole grains, without added refined sugars (check the ingredients list on labels). A "whole grain" consists of 1) the bran, which contains fiber, B vitamins, fats, minerals, and protein; 2) the germ, a source of protein, fats, and vitamins A, B, and E; and 3) the endosperm, which contains complex carbohydrates. Most of the vitamins and minerals in grains are found in their outer layers (the bran and germ), and processing removes both the layers and the nutrients.

A slice of bread or a cup of cooked grain or pasta constitutes one serving.

Eat more complex carbohydrates. In the same vein, you should increase your intake of complex carbohydrates and reduce your intake of simple carbohydrates. Complex carbohydrates are found in unprocessed, unrefined vegetables; in dried beans and peas; in whole wheat products; and in grains including rye, barley, quinoa, millet, brown rice, buckwheat, corn, kamut, and oats. (Remember that white breads, white rice, and many pastas and breakfast cereals have been stripped of most of their complex carbohydrates during processing.)

Simple carbohydrates are mainly in sugars: white and brown sugar, corn syrup, soft drinks, candy, dried fruit, jellies and jams, canned or frozen fruits, ice cream, and pudding. Simple carbohydrates contribute nothing to your diet except calories, and they can upset the way in which the body metabolizes sugar, leading to high blood sugar and adult-onset diabetes. Instead, use unrefined sweeteners such as 100 percent natural maple syrup, honey, and fruit juices. Avoid artificial sweeteners, as research shows they can aggravate diabetes and may cause cancer.

Eat at least 25 grams of fiber daily. Dietary fiber comes from plant cell walls, which our bodies cannot digest. There are two types: insoluble (wheat bran is one example) and soluble, which can be found in oat bran, apples, cherries, and dandelion root, among other foods. A combination of both is recommended to help prevent breast cancer and intestinal diseases such as appendicitis, diverticulosis, and colon cancer.

Eat fish, but curb your intake of other animal products. Red meat, including beef and pork, is associated with increased risk of heart attacks, several forms of cancer, prostate disease, high blood pressure, and a host of other diseases. No more than one serving of red meat per week is recommended.

Chicken and turkey are better for you than red meat, but studies show that ocean fish are far preferable and offer protection against heart disease, multiple sclerosis, cancer, high blood pressure, inflammatory conditions including rheumatoid arthritis, and other diseases. Salmon, mackerel, cod, albacore tuna, halibut, anchovies, and herring are particularly good for you. In general, ocean-caught fish are more healthful than farm-raised fish.

Eat 50 to 150 milligrams of soy isoflavones per day. Soy proteins contain calcium

What Vitamin to Take?

Proper nutrition is the way to support your immune system and prevent disease. However, the diets of most Americans do not meet all of their nutritional needs—and further, scientific research indicates that the optimal level for many nutrients is higher than the Recommended Dietary Allowances (RDA) specified by the Food and Nutrition Board (FNB) of the Academy of Sciences.

Because most people get enough iron from their daily diets, it's generally not necessary to take a multivitamin including iron. If you are pregnant, consult your doctor about the right kind of multivitamin to take. Pregnant women should not take more than 5,000 international units per day of vitamin A, as vitamin A has been shown to cause birth defects in high doses.

I recommend that my patients take a multivitamin daily to get all of the nutrients they need. The following chart shows what a good multiple vitamin/mineral formula should include for adults.

VITAMINS	OPTIMAL RANGE
Biotin	100–300 mcg
Choline	150–500 mg
Folic acid	400–800 mcg
Inositol	150–500 mg
Niacinamide	10–30 mg
Vitamin A (retinol)	5,000–10,000 IU
Vitamin A (from beta-carotene)	5,000–10,000 IU
Vitamin B_1 (thiamin)	10–50 mg
Vitamin B_2 (riboflavin)	10–90 mg
Vitamin B_3 (niacin)	10–90 mg
Vitamin B_5 (pantothenic acid)	100–500 mcg
Vitamin B_6 (pyridoxine)	25–100 mg
Vitamin B_{12}	200–800 mcg
Vitamin C (ascorbic acid)	1,000–6,000 mg
Vitamin D	100–400 IU
Vitamin E (d-alpha-tocopherol)	200–800 IU
Vitamin K (phytonadione)	60–900 mcg

MINERALS	OPTIMAL RANGE
Boron	1–2 mg
Calcium	800–1,200 mg
Chromium	200–400 mcg
Copper	1–2 mg
Iodine	50–150 mcg
Iron	15–30 mg
Magnesium	500–800 mg
Manganese	10–15 mg
Molybdenum	10–25 mcg
Potassium	100–500 mg
Selenium	100–200 mcg
Silica	200–1,000 mcg
Vanadium	50–100 mcg
Zinc	15–45 mg

and plant-derived estrogens, which studies show are effective in preventing osteoporosis and reducing hot flashes in menopausal women. Soy protein can also lower serum cholesterol and reduce the risk of breast, prostate, and colon cancers.

Drink at least eight glasses of water each day to keep your body hydrated. Dehydration causes constipation, dry skin, wrinkles, and kidney problems. It can also impair your ability to concentrate. Filtered water is generally better than public drinking water, which may contain contaminants.

FOODS TO AVOID

It's okay to eat unhealthy foods occasionally. Eating a steak to celebrate a special occasion or indulging in a slice of cake on your birthday will not undermine your immune system and lead to disease. But problems arise when unhealthy eating becomes a habit. Here are some useful guidelines for avoiding foods that, eaten regularly, can compromise your health.

Avoid processed foods. Cooking, canning, peeling, grinding, and other forms of processing tend to destroy disease-preventing nutrients.

Processed foods also have a higher salt and sugar content. Processed and smoked meats, such as luncheon meats, contain nitrates that have been linked to stomach cancer.

Avoid additives, preservatives, and other added chemicals. Additives and preservatives have been shown to aggravate allergies and asthma in sensitive individuals, cause migraine headaches and hyperactivity in children, and possibly cause cancer.

Avoid saturated fats. Foods high in saturated fat contribute to heart disease, adult-onset diabetes, and cancer. Limit your intake of butter, lard, beef, lamb, coconut oil, palm kernel oil, cocoa butter, eggs, cheese, ice cream, and whole milk (skim milk is fine, however). Be sure to distinguish between saturated fats and "good" fats that come from such foods as fish and olive oil.

Avoid too much salt. Eat salt, or sodium chloride, in moderation. Don't add table salt to your food, and avoid salty foods including canned soups and soy sauce. While everyone needs sodium, most of us consume far more than we need. In the United States, the average person consumes between 2,300 and 6,900 milligrams of sodium daily, which is the amount in 1 to 3 teaspoons of salt. The Food and Nutrition Board (FNB) considers 3.5 grams of sodium—about 1 teaspoon of salt—a safe maximum for people not susceptible to high blood pressure. In some people, excess salt leads to fluid retention, which in turn can cause high blood pressure and increase the risk of heart attack, stroke, and kidney damage.

Avoid allergens. Stay away from foods to which you are allergic. Common culprits are dairy products, wheat, corn, peanuts, and citrus fruits. Food allergies can cause a wide range of illnesses and disorders, from headaches and sinusitis to acne, asthma, hives, constipation, joint pain, bron-

chitis, insomnia, and even depression. (See "How to Tell If You Have Food Allergies" on page 26.)

Avoid caffeine. Coffee, colas, and black tea contribute to such nonfatal conditions as insomnia, anxiety, nervousness, dehydration, heart palpitations, high blood pressure, headaches, fatigue, fibrocystic breast disease, nutritional deficiencies, depression, and kidney stones. If you must have caffeine, drink green tea because it also contains other, more healthful ingredients and has been shown to protect against cancer, heart disease, and liver disease.

Avoid alcohol. Alcohol suppresses the immune system and places an enormous strain on the liver. Studies have shown that it can cause high blood pressure and weight gain and can affect blood sugar levels. It has also been linked to an increased risk of breast cancer. Alcoholism is a leading cause of death in the United States.

Avoid tobacco. Tobacco is an even bigger killer than alcohol. Heavy smokers—one pack of cigarettes a day—are four times more likely to die from cancer than nonsmokers. Tobacco is the leading cause of lung, larynx, lip, and esophageal cancer deaths and a significant contributor to bladder, kidney, cervical, pancreatic, and stomach cancers. Cigarettes, cigars, and chewing tobacco are all culprits and should not be used.

THE IMPORTANCE OF EXERCISE

Exercise is just as important as diet. Regular exercise has been shown to reduce blood pressure, reduce cholesterol, reduce obesity, help with insulin metabolism in diabetes, and decrease heart rate. You don't necessarily have to go to a gym every day and build bulging muscles. It's enough just to walk at a fast pace for a half-hour each day,

to stay seated or sit still and may run or climb excessively).

Possible causes include low blood sugar, allergies, learning disabilities, overactive thyroid, and nutritional deficiencies. Taking a B-complex vitamin may be helpful. Hops, lavender, passionflower, and valerian are calming herbs that may also help.

Herbs
Evening primrose
Hops*
Lavender*
Passionflower*
Valerian*

Supplements
Glycine
Omega-3 fatty acids*
Vitamin B_1 (Thiamin)*
Vitamin B_2 (Riboflavin)*
Vitamin B_3 (Niacin)*
Vitamin B_5 (Pantothenic acid)*
Vitamin B_6*
Vitamin B_{12}*
Zinc*

▶ AUTISM

Autism is a disorder that typically results in uneven intellectual development and extreme social withdrawal. People who are autistic lack the ability to form attachments, resist physical contact such as cuddling, and avoid eye contact. They require sameness; they resist change and often engage in rituals, attachment to familiar objects, and repetitive acts. Autism often includes a speech and language disorder that can range from total muteness to a peculiar use of language, with impaired understanding and pronoun reversal, such as using "you" instead of "I."

Autism is associated with deficiencies of nutrients such as folic acid, vitamin B_6, and magnesium.

It may also be related to food allergies, especially sensitivity to sugar, milk, and wheat. Taking a B-complex vitamin and flaxseed oil may be helpful.

Supplements
Folic acid*
Magnesium*
Manganese
Omega-3 fatty acids*
Vitamin B_6*

▶ AUTOIMMUNE DISEASE

An autoimmune disease is one in which, for unknown reasons, the immune system attacks normal parts of the body. Graves' disease, rheumatoid arthritis, lupus, Sjögren's syndrome, polymyositis, dermatomyositis, type 1 diabetes, and multiple sclerosis are some examples of autoimmune disorders. Women are more likely than men to have autoimmune disorders, and relatives of people who have them are often more likely to have the same type of disease. Among people who are already predisposed to a particular disease, a number of factors may provoke its onset. An autoimmune disease may be triggered by a virus, drugs, allergies, or even stress.

For people with autoimmune disease, omega-3 fatty acids may help reduce inflammation and increase the immune response, and a low-fat diet may also boost the immune response.

Supplements
Beta-carotene
Digestive enzymes*
Omega-3 fatty acids*
Omega-6 fatty acids*
Para-aminobenzoic acid
Selenium
Vitamin C*
Vitamin E*

+use supported by Commission E (p. 160)

▶ AUTOIMMUNE THYROIDITIS

In autoimmune thyroiditis, sometimes called Hashimoto's thyroiditis, the immune system attacks the thyroid, inflaming the gland. Some experts believe that this disorder, most prevalent in women between the ages of 30 and 50, is the most common cause of underactive thyroid. People with this condition often have a family history of thyroid disorders. The most frequent symptoms are painless enlargement of the thyroid and a sensation of fullness in the throat. Taking 500 milligrams of tyrosine twice a day may be helpful, since tyrosine is a precursor of thyroxine, a thyroid hormone. If you are taking a thyroid hormone currently, do not take natural products to stimulate the thyroid gland any further, and do not stop any type of synthetic thyroid hormone without consulting your health care provider. Natural products cannot replace synthetic thyroid hormone replacement. If you have an underactive thyroid, get your thyroid hormone levels checked every year by your health care provider.

Supplements
Copper*
Para-aminobenzoic acid
Tyrosine*
Zinc*

▶ BACTERIAL INFECTION

Bacterial infections, which can occur in any part of the body, cause abscesses, carbuncles, pneumonia, diarrhea, strep throat, sinusitis, and any number of other illnesses. The most common types are staphylococcal or streptococcal infections.

Taking antibacterial herbs such as bayberry, garlic, goldenseal, and Oregon grape can be effective for this type of infection. If you have a persistent fever, however, see your doctor as soon as possible.

Herbs
Bayberry*
Chamomile*
Echinacea*
Garlic*
Goldenseal*
Iodine
Oregon grape*

▶ BAD BREATH (HALITOSIS)

Offensive breath can be caused by fermentation of food particles in the mouth, tonsillitis, diabetes, liver disease, sinusitis, gastrointestinal disorders, and dental problems such as cavities or gum disease. In some cases, a deficiency of digestive enzymes may be to blame. Drinking alcohol, smoking, and eating strong foods such as onions and garlic are also frequent causes of bad breath. Some experts recommend eliminating all processed foods, food additives, saturated fats, and sugar from the diet. If you have persistent bad breath, see a doctor to determine the cause.

Herbs
Dandelion
Fennel*
Gentian
Mint*

Supplements
Bromelain*
Digestive enzymes*
Vitamin B$_3$ (Niacin)

▶ BELL'S PALSY

Bell's palsy is numbness of the facial nerve that leads to periodic paralysis on one side of the face. It may also cause pain behind the ear and a feeling of numbness or heaviness in the face; sometimes people with Bell's palsy are unable to close the eye on the affected side. Research shows that injections of vitamin B_{12} are often effective in treating the condition.

Chinese Patent Formula
Da Huo Luo Dan*

Supplement
Vitamin B_{12}*

▶ BENIGN PROSTATIC HYPERPLASIA (BPH)

The condition known as BPH or enlarged prostate is very common in older men, and the incidence increases with age. As the prostate grows larger, it can put pressure on the bladder and urethra (urinary tube), causing a frequent urge to urinate, especially during the night, due to incomplete emptying of the bladder; difficulty starting urination and a decreased urine stream; and dribbling after urination.

One study found that saw palmetto, at a dose of 250 milligrams twice a day, was effective in 90 percent of men with BPH. Eating ¼ cup of zinc-rich raw pumpkin seeds a day is helpful for preventing prostate problems. Studies also show that men who eat tomatoes and tomato products have a decreased risk of prostate cancer, possibly due to the pigment lycopene, which gives tomatoes their red color. Flaxseed oil at a dose of 1 tablespoon a day can help decrease the inflammation of the prostate gland.

Herbs
Pumpkin*
Saw palmetto*
Stinging nettle

Supplements
Alanine*
Copper
Glutamic acid
Glycine
Omega-3 fatty acids*
Zinc*

▶ BILE FLOW OBSTRUCTION

When a blockage or clog occurs in the passageway leading from the liver or gallbladder to the intestine, the flow of bile is obstructed, a condition known as cholestasis. The blockage may be caused by the formation of plugs in the small bile ducts or in the small channel leading to the liver; it can cause jaundice, dark urine, and pale stools. Chronic cholestasis may cause a muddy skin color and bone pain.

Causes of cholestasis include gallstones, alcohol, pregnancy, hormones such as estrogen and oral contraceptives, hepatitis, and certain chemicals and drugs. In people with this condition, blood tests generally show elevated levels of bilirubin, a pigment that helps give bile its greenish yellow color.

One of the functions of bile, which contains cholesterol, lecithin, and bile salts, is to emulsify the fats in foods by breaking them into smaller pieces so they can be digested and absorbed by the small intestine. Herbs that improve bile flow include milk thistle, Oregon grape, wormwood, and yellow dock. These herbs, which tend to be very bitter, can be taken either singly or in combination. In addition, lecithin and digestive en-

*preferred and can be used in combination

zymes help with digestive problems that are often associated with bile flow obstruction.

Herbs
Ginger
Milk thistle*
New Jersey tea
Oregon grape*
Wormwood+
Yellow dock*

Supplements
Digestive enzymes*
Lecithin*
S-adenosylmethionine

▶ BIPOLAR DISORDER

There are two types of bipolar disorder, which is often called manic-depressive disorder. In one type, full-blown manic and major depressive episodes alternate. In the other, periods of depression alternate with shorter periods of mild, nonpsychotic excitement.

During depressive states, people with bipolar disorder may want to sleep all the time and eat constantly. The full-blown manic phase can lead to a dangerously explosive psychotic state in which the person experiences racing thoughts and is impatient, intrusive, and meddlesome, responding with aggressive irritability when crossed. Lack of sleep, hormonal changes, and certain drugs can trigger a manic episode.

It is a good idea to take a daily multivitamin/mineral supplement, since this disorder often causes deficiencies in folic acid, B-complex vitamins, vitamin C, calcium, and omega-3 fatty acids (which you can get by taking 1 tablespoon of flaxseed oil daily). It's important to eat five small meals a day that include some type of protein to help regulate blood sugar levels. Generally, eating

a healthy diet and following a regular exercise program are helpful.

Supplements
Calcium
5-hydroxytryptophan
Folic acid*
Glycine*
Omega-3 fatty acids*
Phenylalanine*
Tryptophan*
Vitamin B$_{12}$*
Vitamin C

▶ BIRTH DEFECTS
See Neural Tube Defects

▶ BLADDER INFECTION

Inflammation of the bladder is usually the result of a bacterial infection. Also known as cystitis, a bladder infection usually causes frequent, urgent, burning, or painful urination, often with frequent nighttime urination and pelvic and back pain. It may make urine cloudy and bloody.

Women are more likely than men to have bladder infections because they have shorter urethras (urinary tubes), which allows bacteria to reach the bladder more easily. Women often get infections after sexual intercourse because bacteria are forced into the urethra and up into the bladder. Using spermicides, perfumed douches, and bubble baths can bring on recurrent infections. Structural problems, particularly in children, can also cause frequent flare-ups. Doctors use urinalysis and urine cultures to diagnose infections.

To prevent recurrent infections, be sure to stay hydrated by drinking eight glasses of water a day. Drinking four glasses of unsweetened cranberry juice daily is another good preventive step, since the juice keeps bacteria from attaching to the bladder wall (cranberry tea is also helpful). Avoid sugar and refined carbohydrates such as white flour because bacteria feed on them, promoting bacterial growth. A bladder infection can move up to affect the kidneys; therefore, if symptoms are not resolved within a day, see a health care provider for diagnosis and treatment.

Herbs that are effective in fighting infections include garlic, goldenseal, grindelia, Oregon grape, raspberry, and uva-ursi, all of which can be used as teas or tinctures. Taking 3,000 milligrams of vitamin C in divided doses (cut back on the total if you experience diarrhea) and 10,000 international units of vitamin A daily will help build up the immune system to fight infections. (See "Winning the Bladder Battle" on page 211.)

Chinese Patent Formulas
- Long Dan Xie Gan Wan
- Shi Lin Tong Pian

Herbs
- Cranberry*
- Echinacea
- Garlic
- Grindelia*
- Goldenseal*
- Goldenrod
- Horsetail
- Juniper*
- Marshmallow
- Oregon grape*
- Pumpkin+
- Raspberry*
- Saw palmetto
- Uva-ursi*

Homeopathic Remedies
- Aconitum napellus
- Apis mellifica
- Berberis vulgaris
- Cantharis
- Mercurius
- Mercurius corrosivus
- Nux vomica
- Pulsatilla
- Sarsaparilla
- Staphysagria

Supplements
- Methionine
- Vitamin A
- Vitamin C*

▶ BLEEDING

Any wound, internal or external, that involves broken skin or blood vessels is likely to bleed. The best way to stop bleeding from an external wound is to apply firm, steady pressure to the area with a clean cloth or bandage. If blood soaks through the compress, add more bandage. If the bleeding doesn't stop within 5 minutes, go to the nearest emergency room; you may have injured an artery or a vein.

If you have had excessive blood loss from a serious injury or surgery, your doctor may order a complete blood count to determine if you have iron-deficiency anemia. If the test shows that you are anemic, the doctor may prescribe iron supplements, but it's not a good idea to take large amounts of iron unnecessarily. Some studies show that iron supplementation may increase the risk of heart disease and cancer.

Homeopathic Remedies
- Aconitum napellus
- Arnica montana
- Bovista
- Carbo vegetabilis
- China officinalis
- Hamamelis
- Ipecacuanha
- Phosphorus*

Supplement
- Iron

+use supported by Commission E (p. 160)

▶ BOILS

Boils, or furuncles, are bacterial skin infections that originate in hair follicles. These painful inflammations occur most frequently on the neck, breasts, face, or buttocks.

To help a boil drain, wet a washcloth, warm it in the microwave (it should be hot but not so hot that it can burn you), and apply it to the boil. Keep the area clean to avoid spreading the infection, wash your hands after touching the boil, and don't share towels or clothing with others. Applying an antibacterial salve containing comfrey, goldenseal, mullein, Oregon grape, or plantain may bring pain relief, and taking vitamins A and C and zinc may help speed healing.

Herbs
Comfrey*
Fenugreek
Goldenseal*
Marshmallow*
Mullein*
Oregon grape*
Plantain*
Tea tree*

Homeopathic Remedies
Arnica montana
Arsenicum album
Belladonna
Hepar sulphuris
Lachesis
Mercurius
Silicea
Staphysagria

Supplements
Vitamin A
Vitamin C
Zinc*

▶ BONE, FRACTURED

See Fractured Bone

▶ BREAST CANCER

Both women and men are susceptible to cancer of the ducts or other cells in the breast, but it is much more common in women. Having a parent, sibling, or child with breast cancer increases the risk by two to three times compared to the risk of people who have no family history of the disease. Other risk factors for women include early onset of menstrual periods, late menopause, first pregnancy after age 30, and a history of certain forms of fibrocystic breast disease in which noncancerous lumps form in the breasts.

To help decrease your risk, eat a diet that's low in fat and sugar and high in soy foods such as soy milk, tempeh, tofu, soy butter, and soy nuts, and add green tea to your beverage list. It may also be a good idea to avoid alcohol, since studies show that drinking even one alcoholic drink a day can increase a woman's risk by up to 30 percent. Regular exercise may be helpful. (See "Reducing Your Risk of Breast Cancer" on page 40.)

To help prevent the formation of free radicals—unstable oxygen molecules in the body that harm healthy cells—and protect against cancer, take a daily multivitamin/mineral supplement that includes antioxidant nutrients such as beta-carotene, selenium, and vitamins A, C, and E. Studies with coenzyme Q_{10} and the hormone DHEA have shown that these supplements may prevent recurrences in women who have had breast cancer. (See "Hormone Replacement Therapy and Breast Cancer" on page 43.)

Since many people discover breast lumps on their own (more than 80 percent of breast cancers are found this way), monthly self-exams are crucial for early detection, as are yearly mammograms after the age of 50.

Herbs
Burdock
Chaparral*
Green tea*

Supplements
Beta-carotene
Coenzyme Q$_{10}$*
DHEA
Melatonin
Omega-3 fatty acids*
Selenium*
Vitamin A*
Vitamin C*
Vitamin D
Vitamin E*

▶ BREASTFEEDING, COMPLICATIONS OF

Since many experts consider mother's milk to be the best food for infants, they recommend breastfeeding for 1 year to prevent allergies. There are health advantages for nursing mothers as well, since studies show that women who breastfeed have a lower risk of breast cancer than women who do not.

Insufficient lactation is decreased production of milk during breastfeeding to the extent that the infant does not receive adequate nutrition. To promote milk production, a mother nursing an infant should change breasts every 10 minutes, four times during each feeding. To help ensure adequate milk, you need to nurse often, drink lots of fluids, eat well, and manage stress. The herbs blessed thistle, dill, fennel, and fenugreek can be used in tincture or tea form to help stimulate breast milk production. Be sure to get 1,200 to 1,500 milligrams of calcium daily when you are breastfeeding.

The easiest remedy for pain caused by a buildup of milk in the breast ducts is simply to nurse more frequently, making sure that the baby empties both breasts at each feeding. Applying warm towels for 10 to 15 minutes before feeding or letting the warm water from a shower flow over your breasts for 15 to 20 minutes will encourage letdown of milk. If your breasts are too full or too hard for your baby to nurse, manually express some milk from each nipple before feeding. Discomfort between feedings can be relieved by applying cold packs to your breasts or armpits. For comfort and support, wear a good nursing brassiere at all times, day and night.

If the nipples become sore, check the position of the baby. Sometimes newborns draw in their lower lip and suck it, which is irritating to the nipple. The mother can ease the lip out with her thumb. Between feedings, the mother can use a hair dryer set on low to warm and dry her nipples for 15 minutes, letting the milk dry on the nipples.

Herbs
Blessed thistle
Dill*
Fennel*
Fenugreek*

Supplement
Calcium*

▶ BREAST TENDERNESS (CYCLIC MASTALGIA)

Many women experience breast soreness or tenderness that occurs a few hours or days before their periods and subsides after menstruation. It is probably related to hormone fluctuations. When breast tenderness, breast cysts, and generalized lumpiness occur together, as they often do, the combination is called fibrocystic breast disease. Taking 1 to 3 grams of omega-6 fatty acids in

*preferred and can be used in combination

Reducing Your Risk of Breast Cancer

More women than ever are developing breast cancer. In 1950, a woman had a 1-in-20 chance of contracting the disease. Today, her chances are 1 in 8. Breast cancer is the second leading cause of cancer death in women aged 40 to 55.

But breast cancer, when detected early, often can be treated. In North America alone, there are more than 2 million breast-cancer survivors. Early detection, early treatment, and a comprehensive program that embraces the best of conventional and complementary therapies offers the best outcome.

No single, definitive cause for breast cancer has been identified. However, various factors are associated with breast-cancer risk.

Family history. A close family member, such as a mother or sister, with breast cancer increases a woman's chance of developing the disease by two to three times. This risk is higher if the relative developed it before menopause.

Early puberty. Menstruation before age 12 creates a 20 percent higher risk of breast cancer, maybe because estrogen has been circulating longer in the woman's system.

Late menopause. Estrogen circulates in a woman's system for a longer period of time.

Delayed childbearing, or having no children. Women who have children before the age of 18 have a reduced risk of breast cancer. Those who have children later or who have no children are at greater risk.

Although some risk factors are difficult to control, certain lifestyle choices have been shown to reduce the risk of breast cancer.

Eat a low-fat diet. Enormous evidence links dietary fat to a variety of cancers, especially breast, colon, and prostate. A diet high in trans-fatty acids, such as vegetable oils, margarine, and red meat, damages healthy cells and may assault the body's genetic material. Also, a high-fat diet stimulates the production of estrogen, which has been implicated in breast cancer.

Drink alcohol in moderation, if at all. Several studies have linked alcohol intake with an increased risk of breast cancer. In one study, published in the *Journal of the American Medical Association* in February 1998, researchers at the

---

the form of capsules or 1 tablespoon of either evening primrose oil or borage oil daily can help reduce tenderness, as can 800 international units of vitamin E and 50 to 100 milligrams of vitamin B$_6$ daily. All of these can be taken together. Eliminate caffeinated beverages such as coffee, black tea, and soda. Cutting out all sugar and saturated fat can also be beneficial.

See also Fibrocystic Breasts

Herbs
Evening primrose

Supplements
Omega-6 fatty acids*
Vitamin B$_6$*
Vitamin E*

▶ BRONCHITIS

Bronchitis is an inflammation of the respiratory passages, usually due to a viral or bacterial infection. Its symptoms include cough, runny nose, fever, chest pain, sore throat, and back and muscle pain. Acute bronchitis is most prevalent

Harvard School of Public Health analyzed six long-term studies involving 320,000 women. They found that women who drank two to five alcoholic drinks a day had a 41 percent greater risk of developing breast cancer than did nondrinkers. Even one drink a day increased breast-cancer risk by 9 percent.

Exercise. A study published in the *New England Journal of Medicine* in May 1997 focused on the link between physical activity and breast-cancer risk. Researchers followed more than 25,000 women for approximately 14 years. They found that those who exercised at least four hours a week had a 37 percent lower risk for developing breast cancer than women who did not exercise.

Decrease the estrogen in your diet. Obesity, a high-fat diet, and excessive consumption of meat, poultry, and dairy products are associated with an increased production of estrogen. Foreign estrogen from pesticides, often found in food, water, and the environment, is a significant contributor to the rise in breast cancer.

Avoid oral contraceptives and hormone replacement therapy. Both have been associated with an increased risk of breast cancer. A study of 918 women, published in the September 1994 issue of the British medical publication *Lancet*, concluded that women who use oral contraceptives for four or more years increase their risk of developing breast cancer at an early age—especially if they begin before age 20. Numerous studies have implicated hormone replacement therapy (HRT) with an increased risk of breast cancer. Fifty-one studies in 21 countries, including more than 52,000 women with breast cancer and another 108,000 who did not have the disease, were combined and analyzed. The results, as reported in a 1997 issue of *Lancet*: The risk of breast cancer increased in women using hormone replacement therapy and in those who used it the longest. Women who used the therapy for 5 or more years had a 35 percent higher risk of developing breast cancer.

Eat soy products. One study reported in *Lancet* showed that women who had a high intake of soy phytoestrogens had a lower risk of breast cancer. This may explain why Asian women have a lower risk of breast cancer. (See "The Soy Solution" on page 250.)

in winter and is often part of an acute upper-respiratory infection. Allergies to pollen, grasses, mold, food, and dust may trigger respiratory inflammation, and chronic bronchitis is very common in smokers.

During a bout with bronchitis, avoid mucus-promoting foods such as milk, cheese, butter, and yogurt, and drink at least eight glasses of water a day. Drinking three or more cups of ginger tea daily can be helpful for cough and congestion. (To make the tea, boil 2 tablespoons of freshly grated ginger in 2 cups of water for 15 minutes, then remove from the heat and steep for 10 minutes.) Since garlic is antibacterial, adding three cloves of raw garlic a day to foods such as vegetables, potatoes, and salad dressings may help bring relief.

You may have a fever of 101° to 102°F for a couple of days, but if it lasts more than 2 days, see your doctor to rule out pneumonia. Clear sputum is a sign of a viral infection or allergy. Try antiviral and antiallergy herbs such as echinacea, horse-

✦use supported by Commission E (p. 160)

radish, licorice, and mullein. Green or yellow sputum indicates a probable bacterial infection, which may benefit from antibacterial herbs such as goldenseal and Oregon grape. Chronic coughs may respond to horehound, licorice, lobelia, mullein, and thyme.

Chinese Patent Formulas

Chuan Bei Jing Pian
Er Chen Wan
Luo Han Guo Chong Ji
Ma Xing Zhi Ke Pian
Ping Chuan Wan
Qing Qi Hua Tan Wan

Herbs

Borage
Comfrey
Echinacea
Elecampane*
Eucalyptus
Garlic*
Ginger*
Ginkgo
Goldenseal
Grindelia*
Horehound
Horseradish
Licorice*
Lobelia*
Mullein*
Mustard
Oregon grape*
Sunflower
Thyme*+
Violet
Wild cherry*

Supplements

Iodine
N-acetylcysteine
Zinc

▶ BRUISES

Bruises, or contusions, are accumulations of blood in tissue underneath the skin. They are usu-ally caused by falls or other physical blows. The typical discoloration of a bruise generally fades within a few days; if it hasn't done so within a week, have a doctor check it.

Nutrients called bioflavonoids strengthen, stabilize, and protect connective tissue and blood vessel walls. You can get these helpful ingredients in blueberries, grapefruit, oranges, cranberries, raspberries, black currants, red grapes, blue plums, cherries, strawberries, and onions. Another way is to take 100 milligrams of the herb bilberry four times a day. Since easy bruising may be a sign of deficiencies of the B vitamins or vitamins C or K, a daily multivitamin/mineral supplement may also be helpful. (Do not take B vitamins separately unless advised to do so by a health care provider, since a high dose of one B vitamin can deplete another.) The number one homeopathic remedy for bruises, sprains, and strains is Arnica montana; beginning as soon after the injury as possible, take three or four 30C pellets every hour for up to three times a day until the pain goes away. It's also a good idea to ice the area as soon and as often as possible to prevent further inflammation.

Herbs

Bilberry*
Boneset
Burdock
Calendula
Comfrey+
Gotu kola*
Juniper
Lavender
Lobelia
Onion
Rosemary
Sage
St. John's wort+
Wormwood

Hormone Replacement Therapy and Breast Cancer

It has been shown that hormone replacement therapy (HRT) may increase a woman's risk of breast cancer.

Ending in 1990, the largest look at women's health in the United States followed 121,700 subjects for 10 years. It found that women who use estrogen alone have a 40 percent greater chance of developing breast cancer than do non-users.

In 1995, concern about the safety of combination estrogen-progestin therapy increased when a follow-up analysis to the above study was published. Researchers found a 40 percent rise in breast cancer among women aged 50 to 64 who had used the combination hormone replacement therapy for 5 years or more, and a 70 percent increase in women aged 65 to 69. The follow-up helped confirm three other European studies which showed similar results.

A team of epidemiologists from the Centers for Disease Control and Prevention and Emory University, both in Atlanta, had similar findings in 1991. The group's meta-analysis of estrogen use from 1976 to 1989 showed a 30 percent increase in the risk of developing breast cancer after 15 years of hormone therapy. Researchers estimated that estrogen use would account annually for about 4,708 new cases of breast cancer and 1,468 deaths from the disease.

Homeopathic Remedies
  Arnica montana
  Bellis perennis
  Hypericum
  Ledum
  Ruta graveolens
  Sulphuricum acidum

Supplements
  B vitamins
  Omega-3 fatty acids*
  Vitamin C*
  Vitamin E*
  Vitamin K*

▶ BURNS

The skin or tissue damage that's caused by burns may be a result of heat, chemicals, or electrical current. In first-degree burns, the skin is not blistered and is red and very sensitive to the touch. Second-degree burns may or may not have blisters; when the burned skin is pressed, it may turn pale and be quite painful. Skin that has suffered a third-degree burn may be black, charred, and leathery but generally does not blister; it may be painless or numb, and hairs can be pulled out easily. It's often hard to distinguish between a deep second-degree burn and a third-degree burn until after 3 to 5 days of observation. There are also fourth-degree burns, which are very deep, involving muscles and nerves. These require emergency medical care. In terms of size, a major burn covers more than 10 to 15 percent of the body surface in children and 25 to 30 percent in adults.

A small burn can be self-treated, but it is very important to keep it clean to avoid infection. Get medical attention for larger burns or those that show signs of infection, including pain, swelling, redness, and pus. The Chinese patent formula Jing Wan Tong is very effective in treating burns. Make sure that the area is clean, then apply the salve and cover with clean gauze. (See "Using Jing Wan Tong to Help Heal Burns" on page 489.) Drink at least eight glasses of water a day to stay hydrated and in-

*preferred and can be used in combination

crease protein intake to help wound healing. Good sources of protein are nuts and seeds, meat, dairy, eggs, and beans. You can apply herbs such as aloe vera, comfrey, gotu kola, St. John's wort, and slippery elm to a new burn and use vitamin E topically later in the healing process to prevent scarring.

Chinese Patent Formula
Jing Wan Tong*

Herbs
Aloe vera*
Burdock
Calendula*
Comfrey*
Gotu kola
Grindelia
St. John's wort+
Slippery elm
Stinging nettle
Tea tree

Homeopathic Remedies
Arnica montana
Cantharis
Causticum
Kali bichromicum
Phosphorus
Urtica urens

Supplements
Isoleucine
Vitamin E

▶ CANCER

In cancer, abnormal changes occur in cells, leading to uncontrolled growth and unusual cellular features. Eventually, a mass forms that can spread to other parts of the body. Cancerous cells often destroy normal cells, resulting in organ failure and loss of function.

Cancers can develop at any age and in any tissue or organ, but, if detected at an early stage, many are curable. In the United States, the incidence of cancer doubles every 5 years after the age of 25. Because of smoking, U.S. lung cancer rates are increasing, and studies show that smokers double their risk of stomach and mouth cancers.

Research shows that taking antioxidant nutrients, including vitamins A, C, and E, and selenium, can protect against cancer. (See "Empowering Your Natural Immunity" on page 253.) Other ways to decrease risk include eating a diet that's low in saturated fat, sugar, and alcohol; eating at least five different fruits and vegetables a day; and exercising 4 or 5 days a week for at least 45 minutes a day.

Studies also suggest that eating soy foods such as tempeh, tofu, soy nuts, soy butter, and soy milk can protect against breast, colon, and prostate cancers. (See "The Soy Solution" on page 250.) Drinking three to five cups of green tea daily may lower risk of stomach, colon, and skin cancers. It may also be helpful to drink filtered water, since tap water can contain lead, bacteria, pesticides, chloride, and many other chemicals.

Cancer patients who receive treatment from an oncologist and a practitioner of natural medicine tend to do better than those being treated solely by conventional medicine. Natural medicine can complement conventional medicine by educating and empowering the patient and enhancing the immune system.

See also Breast Cancer; Colorectal Cancer; Lung Cancer; Skin Cancer; Stomach Cancer

Chinese Patent Formula
Ling Zhi Feng Wang Jiang
Herbs
Asian ginseng
Burdock*
Cascara sagrada*
Chaparral
Garlic*
Green tea
Licorice

Onion
Red clover*
Stinging nettle
Turmeric*

Supplements
Arginine
Glutathione
Melatonin
Quercetin
Selenium*
Shark cartilage
Vitamin A*
Vitamin C*
Vitamin E*

▶ CANDIDA

See Candidiasis, Intestinal; Fungal Infection; Thrush

▶ CANDIDIASIS, INTESTINAL

Intestinal candidiasis is an overgrowth of the yeast *Candida albicans* in the intestines. This overgrowth can cause a variety of both local and body-wide symptoms, such as fatigue, allergic reactions, joint pain, problems with blood sugar regulation, poor memory, a "spacey" feeling, depression, numbness, burning and tingling in the hands and legs, muscle aches, abdominal pain, constipation, diarrhea, bloating, impotence, endometriosis, sugar cravings, headaches, and indigestion. If you have a long history of antibiotic, prednisone (a corticosteroid), or oral contraceptive use (1 month or more) and have some of the symptoms listed, you may have candidiasis.

If you suspect candidiasis, avoid simple carbohydrates, sugars, and yeast-containing foods (breads, alcohol, and dairy products) and see a health care provider for adequate treatment. Anti-

yeast herbs include chamomile, garlic, goldenseal, oregano, pau d'arco, and thyme. Also, it is important to replenish the intestine with good bacteria such as acidophilus, which is found in plain yogurt and in acidophilus capsules and powder, and bifidus, which is available in capsule or powder form.

Herbs
Blue cohosh
Chamomile*
Elecampane
Garlic*
Goldenseal*
Oregano
Oregon grape*
Pau d'arco*
Thyme*

Supplement
Digestive enzymes*

▶ CANKER SORES

Canker sores, also known as aphthous ulcers, are small white mouth ulcers that can be quite painful. The painful phase lasts 3 to 4 days, and symptoms diminish within 7 to 10 days. Attacks can recur two or three times a year, with anywhere from one to several ulcers.

Canker sores occur more frequently in women than in men. Attacks may be triggered by food allergies, chemical sensitivities, or nutritional deficiencies, especially of the B vitamins. (See "Supplements Support Dietary Decisions" on page 311.) Applying tea tree oil topically to the area may relieve the pain, and taking zinc lozenges containing 15 to 50 milligrams of zinc three times a day may help heal the ulcers. Be sure to take 1 to 2 milligrams of copper along with the zinc to avoid copper deficiency, because zinc can inhibit copper absorption.

+use supported by Commission E (p. 160)

Herbs
Chamomile
Echinacea*
Licorice*
Myrrh*
Rose
Tea tree

Supplements
Digestive enzymes*
Folic acid*
Iron
Vitamin B$_1$ (Thiamin)*
Vitamin B$_2$ (Riboflavin)*
Vitamin B$_6$*
Vitamin B$_{12}$*
Zinc*

▶ CAPILLARY FRAGILITY

If capillaries (the smallest blood or lymph vessels) have decreased resistance to physical stress, they become brittle and can rupture or break. Signs of this problem include cramping, decreased circulation, and the appearance of tiny red and blue broken blood vessels in the skin. Foods high in bioflavonoids, including blueberries, grapefruit, oranges, cranberries, red grapes, raspberries, black currants, blue plums, cherries, strawberries, and onion, strengthen, stabilize, and protect the body's connective tissue and blood vessel walls. Eating at least 1 cup a day of these foods can prevent capillary fragility. Or try protective supplements such as bilberry (100 milligrams four times a day), vitamin C (3,000 milligrams a day), and rose hips (100 milligrams three times a day).

Herbs
Bilberry*
Horse chestnut*
Onion
Rose hips*

Supplements
Carnitine
Quercetin
Vitamin C*
Vitamin E*

▶ CARDIOMYOPATHY

Cardiomyopathy is disease of the heart muscle. It causes abnormal enlargement, decreased blood flow, and progressive loss of function, with symptoms such as chest pain, swelling, shortness of breath, and weakness. Coronary artery disease, infections, nutritional disorders, certain drugs, genetic factors, and connective tissue disorders are among the possible causes. People who drink alcohol to excess, have a history of chronically high blood pressure, or have a high-fat diet may be at higher risk for developing cardiomyopathy.

Eating foods that are low in saturated fat and including lots of fruits and vegetables in your diet is a good preventive step. (See "Cut Saturated Fat and Lower Your Risk of Heart Disease" on page 87.) So is exercising at least three times a week for 45 minutes each time. If you have high blood pressure, it's also a good idea to cut back on or eliminate salt.

Herb
Hawthorn*

Supplements
Calcium*
Carnitine
Coenzyme Q$_{10}$*
Magnesium*
Taurine*
Vitamin C
Vitamin E*

▶ CARPAL TUNNEL SYNDROME (CTS)

Carpal tunnel syndrome (CTS) is the name given to the symptoms that occur when excessive repetitive small movements of the hand cause compression of the median nerve in the wrist. People with CTS, the majority of whom are women, have numbness and pain in the wrist, palm, forearm, and shoulder that may be worse at night, and they may have weakness in the thumb, index finger, and forefinger.

Doing yoga strengthening, stretching, and balancing exercises may help reduce pain and improve grip strength. Experts recommend that people who do daily computer work wear a wrist brace, take breaks every hour, and use a specially designed keyboard that allows typing without bending the wrist. They also emphasize proper posture when sitting to prevent constricting nerves in the neck, shoulder, arm, and fingers, and using a chair with proper leg and back support. Vitamin B_6, in the form of 200 milligrams a day of pyridoxine-5-phosphate, is very helpful, and taking 500 milligrams of bromelain and the same amount of quercetin twice a day between meals can help reduce inflammation of the median nerve.

Supplements
Bromelain*
Calcium
Magnesium
Quercetin*
Vitamin B_2 (Riboflavin)*
Vitamin B_6*

▶ CATARACTS

Cataracts, in which progressive clouding of the lens of the eye leads to gradual loss of central vi-sion, are most common in the elderly. The location and extent of the cataract determine how much vision is lost. Although the condition is generally painless, sometimes a cataract causes swelling of the lens that in turn results in glaucoma and causes pain.

Frequent exposure to glaring sunlight and a diet low in antioxidants can increase the risk of cataracts. Research shows that long-term use of high doses of vitamin C (2,000 milligrams or more daily; reduce the dose if you get diarrhea) can substantially reduce the risk, and in one study, supplements of bilberry and vitamin E stopped the progression of cataract formation in 49 out of 50 patients. Other studies show that foods that are high in bioflavonoids, such as blueberries, cherries, strawberries, raspberries, oranges, cranberries, red grapes, black currants, blue plums, onions, and grapefruit, are beneficial to the lens of the eye. Eating ½ cup of these foods daily may reduce the incidence of cataracts. Eliminating dairy products and sugar and eating lots of fruits and vegetables is also helpful.

Herb
Bilberry*

Supplements
Beta-carotene*
Dimethylglycine
Lipoic acid
Quercetin
Selenium*
Vitamin A*
Vitamin B_2 (Riboflavin)*
Vitamin B_3 (Niacin)
Vitamin C*
Vitamin E*
Zinc*

*preferred and can be used in combination

▶ CAVITIES AND TOOTH DECAY

Dental cavities, also known as caries, begin on the external crown or exposed root surface of the tooth. Bacterial plaque, not food debris, causes decay. Cavities begin to form when the plaque is not washed away by saliva or by cleaning methods such as brushing and flossing. The bacteria in the plaque react with sugary and starchy foods to form an acid that dissolves the enamel of the teeth. The damage usually continues unnoticed until symptoms such as sensitivity to heat and cold or discomfort after eating sugary foods signal a problem or a dentist finds decay during a checkup.

The best preventive measures are brushing between meals and flossing daily, rinsing thoroughly after cleaning, and having regular checkups. Since sugary foods and refined carbohydrates such as white bread and crackers tend to stick to the teeth, it's best to avoid them. Studies show that chewing gum that contains xylitol also helps prevent cavities. Fluoride mouthwashes can also help prevent tooth decay.

See also Periodontal Disease

Supplements
Calcium
Xylitol*

▶ CELIAC DISEASE

This chronic intestinal disorder, which causes diarrhea, abdominal discomfort and bloating, weight loss, bone pain, swelling, and skin disorders, is an intolerance to gluten, a protein found in wheat, rye, barley, triticale, and oats. It can occur at any age.

Being diagnosed with this condition (a process that requires an intestinal biopsy) means that you must avoid all foods that contain gluten but may eat products made from grains such as rice, corn, buckwheat, millet, quinoa, and amaranth. Multivitamin/mineral supplements are helpful, since celiac disease may lead to a deficiency of digestive enzymes and fat-soluble vitamins including A, D, E, and K.

Supplements
Bromelain*
Digestive enzymes*
Iron
Vitamin A*
Vitamin D*
Vitamin E*
Vitamin K*

▶ CERVICAL DYSPLASIA

Cervical dysplasia is caused by abnormal cellular changes in the cervix, often as a result of infection by the human papillomavirus (HPV). Untreated, dysplasia can lead to cervical cancer, so regular Pap tests are essential to detect it early.

HPV is not the only cause of dysplasia, however. Studies show that it may be related to deficiencies of beta-carotene, folic acid, selenium, and vitamins A, B_{12}, C, and E. Supplementing with these nutrients in doses of 10 milligrams of folic acid daily (this dose available by prescription only), 50,000 international units of vitamin A a day (dosages this high should be prescribed by a doctor), 6,000 milligrams of vitamin C daily, 400 international units of vitamin E daily, and 200 micrograms of selenium daily may help. A professional practitioner will prescribe 100,000 international units of beta-carotene daily for cervical dysplasia, but such high doses are not recommended without consulting your physician.

the eye, including the iris, the ciliary body, and the choroid), a tumor in the eye, an enlarged cataract, and prolonged use of corticosteroid drugs.

The most common form of glaucoma is chronic open-angle glaucoma. People at higher risk of developing chronic open-angle glaucoma are those with diabetes, high blood pressure, myopia, or a family history of glaucoma. African-Americans have a four to five times greater risk of developing this form of glaucoma than do Caucasians. Symptoms include frequent changes in eyeglass prescriptions, headache, vague visual disturbances, seeing halos around electric lights, and impaired adaptation to the dark. Since glaucoma can have no symptoms until irreversible damage has occurred, routine eye exams are very important. People with severe eye pain and blurred vision should go to the hospital within 12 to 24 hours, because these may be signs of closed-angle glaucoma, which is a medical emergency. Therapy needs to be started as soon as possible to prevent permanent vision loss.

If you have glaucoma, decrease your saturated fat intake, avoid caffeine and alcohol, and eat protein in moderation. A diet high in fruits and vegetables is recommended. Foods high in bioflavonoids, such as blueberries, red grapes, blue plums, raspberries, cherries, strawberries, cranberries, black currants, oranges, grapefruits, and onion, may help protect against glaucoma. Eat ½ cup a day of any of these helpful foods. Individuals with glaucoma should take bilberry (100 milligrams three times a day), an herb that is naturally high in bioflavonoids.

Herb
Bilberry*

Supplements
Chromium
Lipoic acid*
Magnesium
Melatonin
Vitamin A*
Vitamin C*
Vitamin E*

▶ GLOSSITIS

Glossitis is characterized by inflammation, pain, and other changes in the tongue. Pellagra, a niacin (vitamin B$_3$) deficiency, is one cause. This deficiency occurs in areas where Indian corn, or maize, forms a major part of the diet; other symptoms include inflammation of the tissues inside the mouth, diarrhea, dermatitis, and mental aberrations. Other causes include infection, ill-fitting dentures, repeated tongue biting during seizures, alcohol use, tobacco use, hot foods, spices, toothpaste, mouthwashes, breath fresheners, candy dyes, and anemia. A good multivitamin/mineral supplement containing all of the B vitamins is recommended in order to relieve the symptoms of glossitis.

Supplements
Folic acid*
Vitamin B$_2$ (Riboflavin)*
Vitamin B$_3$ (Niacin)*
Vitamin B$_6$*

▶ GOITER

A goiter is an enlargement of the thyroid gland that can be caused by either diminished or excessive thyroid hormone production; excessive ingestion of goitrogens such as turnips, cabbage, brussels sprouts, and broccoli; certain drugs, such as aminosalicylic acid, sulfonylureas, and lithium; and even iodine in large doses. Some goiters are associated with iodine deficiency rather than excess. If you have a goiter in this

*preferred and can be used in combination

category, you should add foods high in iodine, such as kelp, dulse, and hijiki (all from the seaweed family), to your diet. It is important to get an accurate diagnosis for a goiter problem because a thyroid ailment—especially overactive thyroid—can be a medical emergency. Iodine is not recommended unless you have been diagnosed with underactive thyroid. In cases of overactive thyroid, iodine can make the condition much worse.

Herbs
Kelp
Lemon balm

Supplements
Iodine*
Tyrosine

▶ GOUT

Gout, a recurrent arthritis of the peripheral joints, is a condition characterized by excess uric acid, which builds up in the joints, causing bouts of severe pain and inflammation, and can contribute to the formation of uric acid kidney stones. Gout may be triggered by a minor trauma, overindulgence in food or alcohol (especially beer), surgery, fatigue, emotional stress, or infection. Symptoms include joint pain, fever, chills, rapid heart rate, and limited motion in the joints. The pain may last for days or weeks and occurs most often in the big toe, ankle, knee, and elbow joints.

A diet low in foods that contain purines, substances that can trigger uric acid production, has been shown to lower uric acid levels. Foods to avoid include organ meats, red meat, seafood, lentils, beans, peas, alcohol, and sugar. Drinking ½ to 1 quart a day of natural unsweetened cherry juice has been shown to stop the joint pain as-

sociated with gout. Foods high in bioflavonoids, such as blueberries, red grapes, blue plums, raspberries, cherries, oranges, grapefruit, strawberries, cranberries, black currants, and onion, can help reduce inflammation. Eat ½ cup a day of any of these helpful foods. Omega-3 fatty acids such as flaxseed oil (1 tablespoon a day) can help reduce joint inflammation, and a good multivitamin/mineral supplement is recommended as well.

Herbs
Burdock
Chervil
Dandelion
Devil's claw*
Gentian

Supplements
Folic acid*
Omega-3 fatty acids*
Vitamin C*
Zinc*

▶ GROWTH RETARDATION

Growth retardation is a lack of normal growth in a child. Causes of abnormally slow growth and short stature include hypopituitarism, pituitary tumor, growth hormone deficiency, malnutrition, and a condition known as failure to thrive. Inadequate nutrition, the most common cause of growth retardation, can be a result of poverty, poor understanding of feeding techniques, improperly prepared formula, or an inadequate supply of breast milk. A mother who is breastfeeding should take a good multivitamin/mineral supplement. A liquid multivitamin/mineral supplement is recommended for infants and children who are not breastfed.

Supplements
- Biotin
- Calcium*
- Choline
- Iodine
- Iron
- Omega-3 fatty acids*
- Potassium
- Selenium
- Vitamin B$_2$ (Riboflavin)
- Zinc*

Herbs
- Chamomile+
- Green tea*
- Myrrh*
- Sage

Supplements
- Calcium*
- Coenzyme Q$_{10}$*
- Folic acid*
- Vitamin A
- Vitamin C

▶ GUM DISEASE (GINGIVITIS)

Gingivitis is an inflammation of the gums characterized by swelling, redness, and bleeding. It can result from improper brushing or flossing of the teeth to remove plaque. It can also be caused by faulty dental restoration, mouth breathing, diabetes, herpes simplex, use of birth control pills, and exposure to heavy metals such as lead and bismuth. Gum disease is common in puberty and during pregnancy because of the associated hormone shifts.

If you have gum disease, you should eliminate sugar and refined carbohydrates (white-flour products) from your diet. Also, rinsing your mouth daily with a 0.1 percent (1 milligram/milliliter) folic acid solution has been shown to reduce gum inflammation. Supplementation with coenzyme Q$_{10}$ (25 milligrams twice a day) has been shown to reduce the depth and swelling of the gum pockets that occur. People with gum disease also may be deficient in calcium, which should be taken at the recommended dose of 1,200 milligrams a day. (See "Boning Up on Calcium" on page 255.) Daily use of a WaterPik can also be beneficial in preventing gum disease.

▶ HAIR THINNING OR LOSS

Hair thinning or loss can occur on any part of the body as a result of a variety of causes. Hair loss can be attributed to genetic factors, aging, dandruff, psoriasis, a high fever, birth control pills, blood pressure medication, underactive thyroid, syphilis, pregnancy, some drugs, burns, physical trauma, some autoimmune diseases, radiation exposure, and overdoses of vitamin A. Other causes of hair loss are hair dyes, chemicals (such as chlorine in pools), and repeated pulling of the hair.

Male pattern baldness, which has been associated with high levels of testosterone, is the most common form of hair loss. This type of baldness generally starts when a man is in his late thirties, when the hair on the forehead and the top of the head begins to thin and the hairline recedes.

A diet high in fruits and vegetables and low in saturated fat is recommended to boost the immune system, especially if you have one of the diseases listed above that is related to hair loss. You should also take a good multivitamin/mineral supplement that is high in B vitamins. (Do not take B vitamins separately unless advised to do so by a health care provider, since a high dose of one B vitamin can deplete another.) The Chinese

+use supported by Commission E (p. 160)

patent formula Sho Wu Pian has been shown to reverse graying of the hair in some cases and to slow hair loss. The formula should be taken for at least 6 months to obtain the desired results.

Chinese Patent Formula
Sho Wu Pian*

Herbs
Horsetail*
Saw palmetto*
Stinging nettle*

Supplements
Biotin
B vitamins
Copper
Digestive enzymes
Omega-3 fatty acids*
Vitamin B$_2$ (Riboflavin)
Vitamin B$_6$*
Vitamin C
Vitamin E*
Zinc*

▶ HALITOSIS

See Bad Breath

▶ HANGOVER

A hangover is the result of excessive consumption of alcohol, which overwhelms the liver's ability to clear alcohol out of the body. Symptoms are depression, malaise, nausea, headache, irritability, and fatigue the morning after drinking. Digestive enzymes or acidophilus can help relieve these symptoms. Herbs that help detoxify the liver, such as dandelion, gentian, milk thistle, and turmeric, also can be beneficial. Alcohol causes dehydration, so staying hydrated by drinking plenty of water while consuming alcohol can help prevent a hangover.

Herbs
Cayenne pepper
Dandelion*
Gentian*
Milk thistle*
Turmeric*

Supplement
Digestive enzymes

▶ HARDENING OF THE ARTERIES (ATHEROSCLEROSIS)

See Coronary Heart Disease

▶ HARTNUP'S DISEASE

Hartnup's disease is a rare genetic condition in which there is poor absorption of tryptophan and other amino acids. Symptoms include a rash on parts of the body that are exposed to the sun, mental retardation, short stature, headache, and a tendency to collapse or faint. Sunlight, fever, drugs, or other stressors may trigger symptoms. Poor nutritional intake generally precedes the appearance of the symptoms. A diet high in protein is recommended for people with Hartnup's disease because these individuals tend to be deficient in amino acids.

Supplements
Methionine
Niacinamide*
Phenylalanine*
Tryptophan (available by prescription only)*

▶ HAY FEVER

Hay fever is a type of allergic rhinitis affecting the mucous membranes of the eyes and respiratory tract. Causes include pollen from trees such as oak, elm, maple, alder, birch, juniper, and olive; from grasses such as Bermuda, timothy, sweet vernal, orchard, and johnsongrass; and from weeds such as ragweed, Russian thistle, and English plantain.

Allergic reactions generally occur in the spring or fall. Symptoms include itching of the nose and eyes, sneezing, headache, coughing, asthmatic wheezing, red eyes, and clear, watery discharge from the eyes and nose. Hay fever in the spring is often caused by grass and tree pollens, while in the summer or late fall months, it is often caused by weed pollens or mold.

Many people who have severe hay fever symptoms also have food allergies, digestive problems, and nutritional deficiencies. Therefore, eating a whole-foods diet of fresh fruits and vegetables and eliminating any food to which you may be allergic is recommended. Flaxseed oil (1 tablespoon per day) is a natural anti-inflammatory and can help reduce the symptoms associated with hay fever, as can the herb stinging nettle (200 milligrams three times a day). Anti-inflammatory supplements that can help minimize the symptoms associated with hay fever include vitamin C (6,000 milligrams a day; reduce the dose if you get diarrhea), bromelain (500 milligrams twice a day), and quercetin (500 milligrams twice a day).

Hay fever produces a clear, watery nasal discharge, so if you have nasal discharge that is yellow or green it may indicate the presence of a bacterial infection. Pain in the sinus area also can be a sign of a bacterial infection. In either of these cases, see a health care provider.

See also Bacterial Infection

Chinese Patent Formula
Bi Yan Pian

Herbs
Elderberry
Eyebright*
Fenugreek
Grindelia*
Licorice*
Lobelia
Marjoram
Stinging nettle*
White willow

Homeopathic Remedies
Allium cepa*
Arsenicum album*
Euphrasia*
Nux vomica
Sabadilla
Wyethia

Supplements
Bromelain*
N-acetylcysteine
Omega-3 fatty acids*
Quercetin*
Vitamin C*

▶ HEADACHE

Headache can be caused by many factors, including infection, a tumor, a head injury, oral contraceptives, hormonal changes, high blood pressure, tense muscles, anxiety, low blood sugar, emotional tension, sinusitis, allergies, and diseases of the eyes, nose, throat, teeth, and ears.

Headaches that start in the back of the head in the neck area are often due to muscle tension that causes a dull ache that generally becomes worse with movement. Herbs that are helpful for relaxing muscles to relieve a tension headache include chamomile, passionflower, skullcap, and white willow. Eating small, frequent meals can be beneficial for a headache due to low blood sugar. Calcium (1,000 milligrams) and magnesium (500 milligrams) can often relieve a tension headache. If your headache occurs around your eyes and is very painful, causing nausea, vomiting, and

*preferred and can be used in combination

changes in vision, you probably have a migraine. Migraine headaches are often related to food allergies. (See "How to Tell If You Have Food Allergies" on page 26.)

If you have a fever and a stiff neck along with a headache, see a health care provider as soon as possible to rule out meningitis.

See also Migraine

Chinese Patent Formula

Chuan Xiong Cha Tiao Wan*

Herbs

Cayenne pepper*
Chamomile*
Feverfew*
Ginger
Ginkgo
Lovage
Oregano
Passionflower*
Rosemary
Skullcap*
Thyme
Valerian*
White willow*

Homeopathic Remedies

Aconitum napellus
Arnica montana
Belladonna
Bryonia alba
Cocculus
Gelsemium
Glonoinum
Iris versicolor
Kali bichromicum
Lachesis
Natrum muriaticum
Nux vomica
Phosphorus
Pulsatilla
Sanguinaria
Spigelia
Sulphur

Supplements

Calcium
Choline

5-hydroxytryptophan
Magnesium*
Omega-3 fatty acids*
Tryptophan (available by prescription only)
Vitamin B$_2$ (Riboflavin)

▶ HEART ATTACK

A heart attack causes a sudden onset of symptoms related to decreased blood flow to part of the heart. Heart attacks are associated with atherosclerosis, or narrowing of the coronary arteries, which can cause a decrease in blood flow to the heart or a blockage of the artery by a blood clot.

Common symptoms of a heart attack include chest pain that may radiate to the arm, jaw, or shoulder; nausea; anxiety; sweating; shortness of breath; fatigue; and heart palpitations. Taking an aspirin or some white willow bark tincture as soon as possible after a heart attack can prevent further damage. Call 911 immediately if any of these symptoms occur or if you suspect that you or someone else may be having a heart attack. It's crucial to get to a hospital immediately because medication can be given to prevent further damage to the heart.

Diet and exercise are the most important ways to help prevent hardening of the arteries and heart disease. (See "Cut Saturated Fat and Lower Your Risk of Heart Disease" on page 87.) Various herbs and supplements can be used to strengthen the heart and increase oxygen flow to the heart muscle, which can aid recovery from a heart attack. These include hawthorn (100 milligrams per day), coenzyme Q$_{10}$ (50 milligrams per day), taurine (100 milligrams per day), carnitine (500 milligrams per day), calcium (1,000 milligrams per day), and magnesium (500 milligrams per day).

See also Coronary Heart Disease

Herbs
   Hawthorn*
   White willow*

Supplements
   Calcium
   Carnitine*
   Coenzyme Q_{10}*
   Magnesium*
   N-acetylcysteine*
   Selenium*
   Taurine
   Vitamin A*
   Vitamin C*
   Vitamin E*
   Zinc

▶ HEARTBURN

Heartburn is a pain in the chest due to reflux of acid out of the stomach into the esophagus, the passage from the throat to the stomach. Chest pain may radiate into the neck, throat, or even the face. Heartburn generally occurs after meals or when you are lying down. It may be aggravated by smoking or by consuming chocolate, alcohol, tomato products, citrus juices, coffee, peppermint, or spearmint.

Ninety-five percent of those who have heartburn or regurgitation daily to monthly have a hiatal hernia. Avoiding large, fatty meals can help reduce the acid reflux and thus reduce the discomfort of heartburn. To help decrease acid reflux at night, you can eat your main meal early in the afternoon and elevate your head when in bed. Chewable deglycyrrhizinated licorice (400 to 1,200 milligrams chewed 20 minutes before meals) is recommended over licorice tincture in cases of heartburn, hiatal hernia, or peptic ulcer because it is better absorbed, although such a high dose is not recommended without physician supervision because of possible side effects. See

a health care provider to check for esophageal reflux and to get an accurate diagnosis.

Chinese Patent Formula
   Wei Yao*

Herbs
   Aloe vera
   Dandelion
   Horsetail*
   Licorice*
   Oatgrass*
   Slippery elm*

Supplements
   Bromelain*
   Digestive enzymes*

▶ HEART MURMURS

Heart murmurs are abnormal sounds in the heart that can be heard with a stethoscope. They can result from problems with the valves of the heart, the most common of which is mitral valve prolapse. (The mitral valve is the pump between the left ventricle and the rest of the body.) The herbs and supplements listed below can help strengthen the heart muscle and increase oxygen flow to the heart, which can help alleviate symptoms such as shortness of breath. Supplements recommended include calcium (1,000 milligrams per day), magnesium (500 milligrams per day), coenzyme Q_{10} (50 milligrams per day), and carnitine (500 milligrams per day).

See also Mitral Valve Prolapse

Herb
   Hawthorn

Supplements
   Calcium
   Carnitine*
   Coenzyme Q_{10}*
   Magnesium*

+use supported by Commission E (p. 160)

▶ HEAT EXHAUSTION

Exhaustion brought on by intense or prolonged exposure to heat is characterized by profuse sweating with loss of fluids and salts, pale and damp skin, rapid pulse, nausea, and dizziness, all progressing to collapse. Heat exposure combined with dehydration causes heat exhaustion. It is very common in athletes who do not stay hydrated during sporting events.

A person experiencing heat exhaustion should lie down with the feet elevated. Rest is very important. Small amounts of cool, slightly salty water or electrolyte solution (sports drinks such as Gatorade, for example) should be given orally every few minutes.

Homeopathic Remedies
Aconitum napellus*
Apis mellifica
Belladonna
Cuprum metallicum
Gelsemium*
Veratrum album*

Supplement
Sodium

▶ HEATSTROKE

Heatstroke is a disturbance of the temperature-regulating mechanisms of the body caused by overexposure to excessive heat. The symptoms, which include headache, fever, hot and dry skin, and rapid pulse, sometimes progress to delirium and coma. Body temperature can reach 104° to 106°F, and the person feels as if he is "burning up."

Age, obesity, chronic alcoholism, debility, and various drugs, such as anticholinergics, antihistamines, phenothiazines, psychotropic drugs, and cocaine, can increase susceptibility to heatstroke.

To reduce the chance of heatstroke, avoid strenuous exertion, inadequately ventilated areas, and heavy clothing in hot climates or high temperatures. Continuous intake of fluids with salt added is a good idea when you are in very hot climates.

Heatstroke is a medical emergency, so if you suspect that someone is suffering from this condition, call 911 immediately. Remove the person's clothes and try to cool him off with water while waiting for emergency assistance.

Homeopathic Remedies
Aconitum napellus*
Belladonna
Camphora
Gelsemium*
Glonoinum

Supplements
Magnesium*
Potassium*
Sodium*

▶ HEAVY METAL TOXICITY

Heavy metal toxicity is caused by exposure to high amounts of heavy metals such as lead or mercury. Symptoms can include numbness of the legs and feet, high blood pressure, anemia, anxiety, confusion, constipation, depression, fatigue, memory impairment, headache, and pain in the abdomen, bones, and muscles.

The toxic effects of lead can arise from industrial exposure, contaminated water, wine (which may absorb lead from the seal around the cork), mining, smoke inhalation, or gasoline fumes. Mercury can come from dental fillings or contaminated fish. Other heavy metals that can be toxic include aluminum from antacids, deodorants, cookware, and baking soda; cadmium from cigarette smoke; and nickel from stainless steel cookware, super-

Cut Saturated Fat and Lower Your Risk of Heart Disease

Simply put, lowering the amount of saturated fat in your diet reduces your risk of heart disease.

What foods contain saturated fat? Fast foods, fried foods, desserts, dairy products such as eggs and cheese, and red meats are among the top sources. Others include luncheon meats, sausages, hot dogs, and bacon. Also watch for hidden fat in items such as coffee creamers, whipped toppings, and dips.

Try to keep total fat consumption to 20 percent or 25 percent of calories. Most Americans eat up to 40 percent of calories from fat. A gram of fat contains 9 calories; a gram of carbohydrate or protein has only 4 calories. So, eating fat puts on the fat.

Saturated is the most detrimental kind of fat. Healthful fats are found in certain oils, including cold-pressed canola and walnut, and in fresh raw nuts and seeds such as almonds, walnuts, pecans, cashews, and sunflower and pumpkin seeds. Studies have shown that eating nuts can reduce cholesterol levels and the risk of fatal heart attack.

You can lower saturated fat in your diet by opting for lean proteins such as chicken without the skin, fish, and legumes such as dried peas and beans.

When choosing meats, look for lean cuts and trim excess fat. Remember, though, that lean cuts of beef contain fat even after trimming. Use a fat separator or strainer when making gravies and soup stocks.

When it comes to dairy products, select skim milk, fat-free yogurt, and fat-free cheese over regular products. Substitute egg whites for whole eggs. (Use two egg whites for every whole egg when baking, for example.) Limit egg yolks to one per serving when cooking scrambled eggs, and add egg whites for larger servings. Instead of frying, try low-fat cooking options such as steaming, boiling, baking, and broiling, and use a nonstick pan or cooking spray.

If you fry or sauté foods, be aware that even healthful oils are damaged by heat. An oil is breaking down if it smokes during cooking. To minimize breakdown, cook at the lowest heat possible and choose an oil, such as olive, canola, or sunflower, that is less vulnerable to deterioration.

---

phosphate fertilizers, and tobacco smoke. A hair mineral analysis can be used to detect heavy metal toxicity. See a health care provider for detoxification recommendations if you suspect that you have toxicity. The remedies listed below can help chelate the heavy metals out of the body.

Herbs
Dandelion
Milk thistle
Turmeric

Supplements
Choline*
Cysteine*
Methionine*
Vitamin C

▶ HEMORRHOIDS

Hemorrhoids are enlarged, dilated veins in the anus or rectum that produce visible bulges and sometimes pain and bleeding. Hemorrhoidal bleeding typically occurs following bowel movements and is evident on toilet tissue. (Any blood noted in the stool should be reported to your health care provider, because blood in the stool can be a sign of colon cancer.)

*preferred and can be used in combination

Herbs

Black cohosh*+
Blessed thistle
Blue cohosh*
Chamomile
Dandelion
Dong quai (Dang gui)*
Evening primrose
Feverfew*
Gentian
Lemon balm
Lovage
Mint
Rose hips
Thyme
Turmeric*
Valerian*
Wild yam*
White willow*
Yarrow+

Homeopathic Remedies

Belladonna
Chamomilla
Colocynthis
Nux vomica
Pulsatilla

Supplements

Calcium
Magnesium
Omega-3 fatty acids*
Omega-6 fatty acids
Vitamin B₆*

▶ MENSTRUAL PERIODS, LACK OF (AMENORRHEA)

The absence of menstrual periods may be related to psychological disturbances, diet and exercise habits, lifestyle, environmental stresses, a family history of genetic problems, polycystic ovarian syndrome, hormone imbalances, or abnormal growth and development. Lack of menstruation due to overexercising, eating disorders, or nutritional deficiencies can increase the risk of osteoporosis.

Naturally, lack of menstruation is normal before puberty, during pregnancy and nursing, and after menopause. (See "Signs and Symptoms of Menopause" on page 111.) Otherwise, however, it is important to get an accurate diagnosis if you miss your period for more than 2 months, so see a doctor. He or she will first test for possible pregnancy. Taking herbs during pregnancy can harm the fetus. Therefore, do any take any of the remedies below without professional guidance.

Chinese Patent Formula

Bu Xue Tiao Jing Pian

Herbs

Black cohosh*
Blue cohosh
Calendula
Licorice*
Madder
Rue
Wild yam*

Supplements

Calcium
Magnesium

▶ MIGRAINE

A migraine is a severe head pain related to abnormal dilation of blood vessels in the head that is sometimes preceded by warning signs such as visual disturbances and is often accompanied by symptoms such as sensitivity to light or sound, depression, restlessness, and nausea and vomiting. Migraine headaches generally start on one side of the face or head.

Migraines are often associated with food allergies, especially to tyramine-containing foods such as chocolate, cheese, beer, sour cream, fer-

+use supported by Commission E (p. 160)

mented sausages, aged meats, chicken liver, wine, and yeast-containing foods. Other foods that have been associated with migraines include food coloring and flavoring agents, coffee, tea, aspartame, milk, monosodium glutamate (MSG), and nitrates from hot dogs and cured meats.

Other factors that can trigger migraines include stress; low blood sugar; infections of the eyes, ears, teeth, or sinuses; and head injury. If you are prone to migraines, you should have some allergy tests or try an elimination diet to determine if you have any food sensitivities that might be triggering headaches. (See "How to Tell If You Have Food Allergies" on page 26.) Natural anti-inflammatory herbs such as cayenne pepper, feverfew, skullcap, valerian, and white willow can also be helpful.

Chinese Patent Formula
Tian Ma Wan

Herbs
Cayenne pepper

Feverfew*

Skullcap

Valerian

White willow*

Supplements
Calcium*

5-hydroxytryptophan*

Magnesium*

Omega-3 fatty acids*

Quercetin*

Vitamin B_2 (Riboflavin)*

Vitamin B_3 (Niacin)

▶ MISCARRIAGE, THREATENED

A threatened miscarriage is the possibility of a spontaneous abortion. Bleeding can be a sign of a miscarriage or threatened miscarriage. For a woman who has had repeated miscarriages, taking

omega-3 fatty acids (1 tablespoon of flaxseed oil a day) or omega-6 fatty acids (1 to 3 grams in capsule form or 1 tablespoon daily of black currant, borage, or evening primrose oil) throughout pregnancy can be beneficial. Raspberry tea (two to three cups a day) is often used throughout pregnancy to strengthen the uterus. If you experience any vaginal bleeding during pregnancy, see a health care provider as soon as possible.

Chinese Patent Formula
An Tai Wan*

Herb
Raspberry*

Supplements
Omega-3 fatty acids*

Omega-6 fatty acids

▶ MITRAL VALVE PROLAPSE

This is a common heart disorder in which the mitral valve—the pump between the left ventricle and the rest of the body—protrudes into the left ventricle. People with this condition are usually symptom-free, but some may experience palpitations, fainting, fatigue, and chest pain. A heart murmur is commonly heard in people with this condition.

A carnitine deficiency has been suggested as a causative factor for mitral valve prolapse. Coenzyme Q_{10} at a dose of 10 to 50 milligrams per day has been shown to be effective in children ages 8 to 16 with symptomatic mitral valve prolapses. See your health care provider for an accurate diagnosis.

Supplements
Calcium*

Carnitine*

Coenzyme Q_{10}*

Magnesium*

▶ MONONUCLEOSIS

Mononucleosis, also known as the kissing disease, is transmitted by secretions from the mouth and nose. It is caused by a type of herpesvirus known as Epstein-Barr. Symptoms include fatigue, weakness, mild fever, swollen lymph glands, and a sore throat. It is most often seen in young adults.

Mononucleosis generally lasts from 2 to 6 weeks. In rare and severe cases, it can have some serious complications, such as seizures, spleen and liver enlargement, and numbness in the legs and feet. If you have mononucleosis, it is important to follow a good diet, get plenty of rest, and stay hydrated. Herbs that stimulate the immune system include echinacea, garlic (three raw cloves a day), ginger, and licorice. A good multivitamin/mineral supplement is recommended. Ginseng (Asian or Siberian) helps boost the immune system and increase energy levels. (See "Herbal Immune-Boosters" on page 162 and "Empowering Your Natural Immunity" on page 253.)

Herbs
Asian ginseng
Echinacea*
Garlic*
Ginger*
Goldenseal
Licorice*
Marshmallow
Oregon grape*
Siberian ginseng*

Supplements
Vitamin A*
Vitamin C*
Zinc*

▶ MONOSODIUM GLUTAMATE (MSG) INTOLERANCE

People who have monosodium glutamate intolerance are unable to consume monosodium glutamate (MSG), a flavor enhancer found most commonly in Chinese food, without developing an allergic-type reaction. The allergic reaction can be hives, shortness of breath, a hot and flushed feeling, or other symptoms. Vitamin B_6 has been shown to reduce this allergic-type reaction in some people.

Supplement
Vitamin B_6*

▶ MORNING SICKNESS

Morning sickness, often experienced by women in the first trimester of pregnancy, is characterized by early-morning nausea and/or vomiting. It is a common condition that usually resolves itself, but it can become a serious problem if it continues beyond 3 months of pregnancy or becomes quite frequent, because the nausea can prevent a woman from eating.

Causes of morning sickness include the increasing levels of hormones, liver congestion, decreased hydrochloric acid in the stomach, emotional stress, and changes in carbohydrate metabolism. Eating small, frequent meals of foods such as crackers or toast, especially before getting up in the morning, may help reduce nausea and vomiting. Ginger tea is also recommended. To make the tea, boil 2 tablespoons of grated fresh ginger in 2 cups of water for 15 minutes, then remove from the heat and steep for 10 minutes. (See "Ipecacuanha for Nausea and Vomiting in Pregnancy" on page 414.)

---

*preferred and can be used in combination

Herbs
Chamomile*
Ginger*
Raspberry
Star anise*

Homeopathic Remedies
Antimonium crudum
Antimonium tartaricum
Arsenicum album
Belladonna
Cocculus
Colocynthis
Ipecacuanha
Nux vomica
Petroleum
Phosphorus
Tabacum
Veratrum album

Supplements
Bromelain*
Chromium
Digestive enzymes*
Vitamin B$_6$*
Vitamin C
Vitamin K

▶ MOTION SICKNESS

Motion sickness is the nausea and sometimes vomiting caused by rhythmic movement such as that experienced when riding in a car or boat. Eating pumpkin and squash seeds has been shown to prevent and alleviate motion sickness, as have the wrist acupressure bracelets that are available in many drugstores. Ginger is also helpful for alleviating nausea. To make a tea, boil 2 tablespoons of grated fresh ginger in 2 cups of water for 15 minutes, then remove from the heat and steep for 10 minutes. Candied ginger is also effective and is convenient if you are in an area where hot water is not available to make tea.

See also Nausea

Chinese Patent Formula
Ren Dan

Herb
Ginger*+

Homeopathic Remedies
Antimonium crudum
Antimonium tartaricum
Arsenicum album
Belladonna
Cocculus
Colocynthis
Ipecacuanha
Nux vomica
Petroleum
Phosphorus
Tabacum
Veratrum album

▶ MOUTH IRRITATION

Mouth irritation or inflammation can be caused by such things as canker sores, a cut, gum disease, or poorly fitted dentures. A mouthwash that includes myrrh, sage, or tea tree can be helpful. If the irritation does not go away within a couple of days, see a dentist.

See also Canker Sores; Gum Disease

Herbs
Myrrh*
Sage
Tea tree*

▶ MULTIPLE SCLEROSIS (MS)

Multiple sclerosis (MS) is an autoimmune disease in which the immune system attacks the central nervous system, causing intermittent attacks of muscular and sensory symptoms and, often, progressive disability. Symptoms, which can be unpredictable and intermittent, include numbness and weakness in one or more extremities, visual disturbances such as blindness, difficulties with bladder control, memory loss, fatigue, slurred speech, and vertigo or dizziness. Some people may have only one attack of MS, while others may have recurrent attacks, with symptoms worsening as time goes on.

Multiple sclerosis is most common in women between the ages of 20 and 45. While the exact cause is unknown, some researchers believe that it can be the result of a viral infection, an autoimmune disease, heavy metal toxicity, or food allergies. A low-fat diet that provides 10 to 15 grams of fat a day has been shown to improve energy and fatigue levels in people with multiple sclerosis. Deficiencies of vitamin B_6 and B_{12} have also been associated with MS. Supplementation with omega-3 fatty acids (1 tablespoon of flaxseed oil a day) and omega-6 fatty acids (1 to 3 grams in capsule form or 1 tablespoon per day of black currant, evening primrose, or borage oil) have been shown to slow the progression of the disease.

Deficiencies of some vitamins and minerals, including calcium, magnesium, selenium, vitamin D, and zinc, have been shown to cause a predisposition to MS. If you have multiple sclerosis, take a good multivitamin/mineral supplement; avoid all processed foods, food additives, preservatives, colorings, flavorings, caffeine, tobacco, and alcohol; and eat only fresh, unprocessed foods. In addition, exercise is important to keep energy levels high.

Herbs
Asian ginseng
Ginkgo*
Siberian ginseng*

Supplements
Calcium*
Digestive enzymes*
Magnesium*

Omega-3 fatty acids*
Omega-6 fatty acids
Selenium*
Vitamin B_6*
Vitamin B_{12}*
Vitamin C*
Vitamin E*
Zinc

▶ MUMPS

Mumps is an infectious viral disease characterized by inflammation and swelling of the parotid gland and other salivary glands and sometimes by inflammation of the testes or ovaries. It is caused by a paramyxovirus. Symptoms include headache, fever, fatigue, and muscle weakness and pain.

Mumps is spread by droplets dispersed from the nose, throat, and mouth by coughing or sneezing and by direct contact with objects contaminated by infected saliva. The incidence of mumps peaks in late winter and early spring, and most cases occur in children ages 5 to 15. Mumps can be contagious from 1 week before the onset of the disease to 2 weeks afterward. One episode of mumps gives lifelong immunity.

People with mumps should rest, drink plenty of fluids, and eat healthy foods. Nutrients that help build up the immune system include echinacea, garlic, ginger, selenium, vitamins A and C, and zinc.

Herbs
Echinacea*
Garlic*
Ginger*

Homeopathic Remedies
Aconitum napellus
Apis mellifica
Arsenicum album
Belladonna
Bryonia alba
Carbo vegetabilis

+use supported by Commission E (p. 160)

Mercurius
Phytolacca
Pilocarpus jaborandi
Pulsatilla
Rhus toxicodendron

Supplements
Selenium*
Vitamin A*
Vitamin C*
Zinc*

▶ MUSCLE CRAMPS

See Leg Cramps

▶ MUSCLE STRAIN

A strain is an injury to a muscle, generally in the lower back, from overuse or improper use. Strains commonly occur in people who participate in sports that require pushing or pulling against resistance, such as weight lifting or football (for example, pushing against an opposing lineman). They can also occur in sports that require twisting of the back, such as basketball, baseball (swinging a bat), or golf (swinging a club). Symptoms include sudden back pain while twisting, pushing, or pulling. Stop the activity immediately if you start to feel such pain; do not overexert yourself by trying to finish the game.

If you get a muscle strain, use the PRICE (protect, rest, ice, compress, and elevate) treatment as soon as possible. Taking the homeopathic remedy Arnica montana (3 to 4 pellets of arnica 30C each hour at least 20 minutes before or after taking any food or drink until the pain resolves) is very effective for muscle sprains, strains, and bruises. (See "Natural Therapies for Sprains and Strains" on page 146.)

It is very important to decrease inflammation, because inflammation to the area can cause fur-

ther injury. Natural anti-inflammatories include feverfew, passionflower, turmeric, white willow, bromelain, calcium, magnesium, and quercetin.

Chinese Patent Formulas
Die Da Wan Hua You
Zhui Feng Huo Xue Pian

Herbs
Feverfew
Kava kava+
Passionflower
St. John's wort+ (external)
Turmeric
White willow
Wintergreen

Homeopathic Remedies
Arnica montana*
Rhus toxicodendron

Supplements
Bromelain*
Calcium*
DMSO
Magnesium*
Quercetin*

▶ MUSCULAR DYSTROPHY

Muscular dystrophy refers to any of several genetic conditions that lead to progressive weakness of muscles. Symptoms include muscle weakness that causes toe walking, frequent falls, and difficulty in standing up and climbing stairs. Duchenne type muscular dystrophy is a recessive disorder that is linked to the X chromosome. The disease is most common in boys ages 3 to 7. Becker's muscular dystrophy is also an X-linked disorder that occurs in children. There are several other muscular dystrophy disorders that are not discussed here.

Studies show that coenzyme Q_{10}, selenium, and vitamin E may be beneficial for muscular dystrophy. Glutamine may be beneficial in children with Duchenne type muscular dystrophy because it has been shown to decrease degradation of body protein. Creatine has been shown to prevent further muscle weakness.

Chinese Patent Formula
Jian Bu Hu Qian Wan

Supplements
Coenzyme Q_{10}*
Creatine*
Glutamine
Selenium*
Vitamin E*

▶ MUSHROOM POISONING

The death cap mushroom contains a poison called phalloidin. Within 6 to 24 hours of eating the mushrooms, symptoms of poisoning occur, including excessive salivation, sweating, vomiting, abdominal cramps, diarrhea, confusion, coma, and occasionally convulsions. Jaundice due to liver damage is common and develops in 2 to 3 days. While recovery is possible, the death rate is greater than 50 percent, with death occurring in 5 to 8 days. The potential for poisoning by mushrooms is unpredictable; it may vary within the same species, at different times of the growing season, and with cooking. Milk thistle and lipoic acid may be used as mild antidotes, but to be safe, you should never experiment with mushrooms in any form. Do not try to self-treat mushroom poisoning. If you do get sick from any type of mushroom ingestion, go to the nearest emergency room as soon as possible.

Herb
Milk thistle*

Supplement
Lipoic acid

▶ MYASTHENIA GRAVIS

Myasthenia gravis is an autoimmune disease in which the muscles are attacked by the immune system, leading to muscle weakness and severe fatigue. The condition is caused by blocked or damaged acetylcholine receptors that control muscle activity. This disease occurs in women, predominantly between the ages of 20 and 40, but it can occur at any age. Symptoms include drooping eyelids, double vision, and severe muscle weakness after exercise. Other symptoms include difficulty walking, difficulty speaking, and problems lifting or holding objects. A healthy diet and exercise program is recommended to help the condition. Creatine may prevent further muscle weakness.

Supplements
Calcium
Choline*
Creatine
Magnesium
Manganese*
Omega-3 fatty acids*
Vitamin B_6*

▶ NARCOLEPSY

Narcolepsy is a genetic condition in which the affected person can suddenly fall asleep at any time of the day or night. The exact cause is unknown. Symptoms, which begin in adolescence and persist throughout life, include sleep attacks, lasting from a few minutes to several hours, that range from a few a day to many a day. Visual illusions or hallucinations may occur at the onset of sleep.

Eating small, frequent meals with protein at each meal can help regulate blood sugar imbalances that may be associated with narcolepsy. A good multivitamin/mineral supplement that in-

*preferred and can be used in combination

cludes all the B vitamins is also recommended. (Do not take B vitamins separately unless advised to do so by a health care provider, since a high dose of one B vitamin can deplete another.) Tyrosine may be deficient in people who have narcolepsy and thus may be useful as a supplement, and Siberian ginseng may help to boost both the immune system and energy levels.

Herbs
    Asian ginseng
    Siberian ginseng*
Supplements
    B vitamins
    Tyrosine*

▶ NAUSEA

Nausea is the unpleasant sensation in the stomach that often precedes vomiting. Nausea and vomiting may be associated with motion sickness, pregnancy, viral infection, migraine headache, a drug reaction, anxiety, or intestinal bacterial infection. Ginger tea is very beneficial for nausea. To make it, boil 2 tablespoons of grated fresh ginger in 2 cups of water for 15 minutes, then remove from the heat and steep for 10 minutes. Eating crackers and frequent small meals may also help reduce nausea. If vomiting persists for more than an hour, it may be the result of a bacterial infection from food poisoning, especially if there is also diarrhea. Please see your health care provider for persistent vomiting and nausea in order to get an accurate diagnosis.

See also Angina; Anxiety Attacks; Cholecystitis; Crohn's Disease; Dysentery; Dyspepsia; Food Poisoning; Gallstones; Gastritis; Hangover; Headache; Heart Attack; Heat Exhaustion; Hepatitis; Indigestion; Jaundice; Kidney Stones; Lupus; Migraine; Morning Sickness; Motion Sickness; Mushroom Poisoning; Peptic Ulcer; Pregnancy Complications; Radiation Exposure; Renal Failure; Stomach Cancer; Whooping Cough

Herbs
    Chamomile*
    Gentian
    Ginger*
    Mint
    Raspberry*
Homeopathic Remedies
    Antimonium crudum
    Antimonium tartaricum
    Arsenicum album
    Belladonna
    Cocculus
    Colocynthis
    Ipecacuanha
    Nux vomica
    Petroleum
    Phosphorus
    Tabacum
    Veratrum album
Supplements
    Bromelain*
    Digestive enzymes*

▶ NERVOUSNESS

Nervousness is excessive irritability that is accompanied by mental and physical unrest. It can be a result of drinking too many caffeinated beverages, low blood sugar, high blood sugar, overactive thyroid, and many other health conditions. Foods that help strengthen the nervous system and are calming include oats, nuts, seeds, poultry, and red meats.

If you are constantly nervous, it may indicate that you are lacking in B vitamins. The best way to take them is in a B-complex vitamin that contains 1,000 micrograms of vitamin B_{12} and all the other B vitamins in 50-milligram doses. (Do not take B vitamins separately unless advised to do so by a health care provider, since a high dose of one B vitamin can deplete another.) Calming herbs that can be taken as tea or tincture include catnip, chamomile, hops, passionflower, skullcap, and valerian. Please see your health care provider to get an accurate diagnosis.

Herbs
Catnip*
Chamomile*
Hemlock
Hops*
Passionflower*
Skullcap*
Valerian*

Supplement
B vitamins

▶ NEURALGIA AND NEURITIS

Neuralgia is nerve pain generally associated with neuritis, an inflammation of a nerve, often marked by pain, numbness, tingling, or paralysis, generally in the hands, arms, legs, and feet. Deficiencies of vitamin B_{12}, vitamin B_1 (thiamin), folic acid, and vitamin E have been associated with neuralgia, so supplements of these vitamins may help relieve the condition. Vitamin B_6 can cause numbness and a tingling in the legs or hands at a dose as low as 200 milligrams a day; pregnant women should not take more than 100 milligrams a day (consult a physician).

Coenzyme Q_{10} may also be helpful for increasing oxygen and circulation to the area. A salve of cayenne pepper, horseradish, and peppermint applied over the area of the pain can be soothing.

Herbs
Cayenne pepper*
Devil's claw+
Horseradish

Mint+
White willow

Supplements
Bromelain
Coenzyme Q_{10}
Folic acid
Omega-3 fatty acids*
Quercetin
Vitamin B_1 (Thiamin)*
Vitamin B_{12}*
Vitamin E*
Zinc*

▶ NEURAL TUBE DEFECTS

Neural tube defects are a developmental abnormality resulting in anencephaly or spina bifida. These birth defects may be prevented if the mother takes a good prenatal vitamin containing folic acid (800 micrograms a day) throughout her pregnancy. Other possible causes of neural tube defects in infants include malnutrition of the mother while pregnant and alcohol or drug use during pregnancy. Ideally, women who want to become pregnant should begin taking a prenatal vitamin even before conception.

Supplements
Folic acid*
Zinc*

▶ NIGHT BLINDNESS

Night blindness is a condition in which vision is normal in daylight but abnormally poor in dim light or at night, possibly due to a vitamin A or zinc deficiency. Conditions that may cause a vitamin A or zinc deficiency include malnutrition, celiac disease, cystic fibrosis, surgery on the pancreas and/or duodenum, giardiasis, and cirrhosis of the liver. Night blindness can also be a sign of

+use supported by Commission E (p. 160)

cataracts, macular degeneration, glaucoma, or retinitis pigmentosa.

To get more vitamin A in your diet, eat foods such as fish-liver oils (1 tablespoon per day of cod-liver oil) and egg yolks. Be careful not to consume too much vitamin A. Signs of vitamin A overdose include hair loss, joint pain, muscle pain, and fatigue. Eating ½ cup a day of foods high in bioflavonoids, such as blueberries, cherries, strawberries, raspberries, oranges, cranberries, red grapes, black currants, blue plums, onion, and grapefruit, may help improve blood flow to the eyes. Bilberry (100 milligrams three times a day) is also a natural bioflavonoid. The Chinese traditionally believe that vision problems can be related to a congested liver. (See "Healthy Living Starts with a Healthy Liver" on page 462.)

Chinese Patent Formulas
Qi Ju Di Huang Wan

Ming Mu Di Huang Wan

Herb
Bilberry*

Supplements
Beta-carotene

Omega-3 fatty acids*

Vitamin A*

Zinc

▶ OBESITY

Obesity is defined as being 20 percent or more over the ideal weight listed on standard height-weight tables for the relevant height and frame. People who are 20 to 40 percent overweight are classified as mildly obese; 41 to 100 percent overweight, moderately obese; and more than 100 percent overweight, severely obese. Obesity can increase the risk of coronary heart disease, diabetes, stroke, high cholesterol, and high blood pressure.

Fad diets are generally unsuccessful because within the first year off the diet, people usually regain whatever weight they lost while on the diet. The best way to lose weight is with a program of exercise and healthy eating. The diet should be low in sugar, high in fiber (including fruits and vegetables), and low in saturated fat. If you need to lose weight, eat only fresh, non-processed foods with no preservatives or artificial flavorings. A rule of thumb is that if a food comes in a package, can, or box, it probably has been processed and therefore is not healthy for you.

Have your main meal at lunchtime and avoid eating late at night. (See "Tried and True Tips for Losing Weight.") Nutrients that help reduce sugar cravings include chromium and gymnema. Omega-3 fatty acids (1 tablespoon daily of flaxseed oil) actually help to metabolize fat.

Chinese Patent Formula
Bojenmi Chinese Tea*

Herbs
Guaraná

Gymnema*

Kelp

Psyllium

Supplements
Chromium*

5-hydroxytryptophan*

Omega-3 fatty acids

Pyruvate*

S-adenosylmethione*

Vitamin B$_5$ (Pantothenic acid)

▶ OSGOOD-SCHLATTER DISEASE

Osgood-Schlatter disease is an inflammation and soreness of the knee joints. It occurs in boys between the ages of 10 and 15, perhaps caused by

Tried and True Tips for Losing Weight

If you want to lose weight, don't set yourself up for failure. Instead, set a realistic target—usually a loss of 1 or 2 pounds a week. To achieve your goal, try these tips:

- Get to know your problem eating habits. Keep a food diary for a week or two, writing down everything you eat. This will heighten your awareness of high-calorie snacking, mood-related eating, and weekend lapses.
- Avoid temptation—don't keep high-calorie foods on hand. A calorie chart can help identify loaded foods.
- Cut out high-calorie foods such as sugar, alcohol, and fat-filled butter, cream, cheese, salad dressings, red meats, cakes, and pastries.
- Use low-calorie spices such as garlic, basil, oregano, and ginger to perk up foods, instead of calorie-laden gravies and cream sauces.
- Fill up on fruits and vegetables. They're higher in nutritive value and lower in calories.
- Plan meals so you don't binge. And don't eat while watching television, when you may not realize how much food you're tucking away.
- Instead of giving up favorite foods, eat smaller portions, which also helps put the brakes on bingeing. A portion should be about the size of a woman's palm.
- Chew your food at least 20 times per forkful. You'll digest it better—and give your stomach time to signal when it's full.
- Exercise. Aim for 45 minutes or more at a time, three to six times a week. Options include walking, hiking, running, swimming, cross-country skiing, bicycling, aerobics, and yoga.
- Don't feel guilty if you slip now and then. Just get back on track.
- Above all, believe in yourself. You can and will succeed.

trauma to the knees. Symptoms include pain, swelling, and tenderness in the knee that tends to be worse when walking down stairs or down a hill. Vitamin E (400 international units a day) and selenium (200 micrograms a day) have been shown to prevent Osgood-Schlatter disease.

Supplements
Selenium*
Vitamin E*

▶ OSTEOARTHRITIS

Osteoarthritis is a degenerative joint disease that affects many people from age 40 on and is marked by chronic breakdown of cartilage in the joints that leads to pain, stiffness, and swelling. It is also called degenerative joint disease or wear-and-tear arthritis. The joints most affected are those of the knees, hips, neck, and lower back. As a joint begins to wear with age, the cartilage also wears down, causing pain and inflammation. Most people over age 50 have some degree of osteoarthritis.

Rest, elevating the legs, and icing the affected area may help inflammation and pain. Eliminating the nightshade vegetables—tomatoes, white potatoes, tobacco, eggplant, and green, yellow, and red peppers—from your diet may also help reduce the pain and swelling. Eating ½ cup a day of foods high in nutrients called bioflavonoids,

*preferred and can be used in combination

which are found in high concentrations in foods such as blueberries, cherries, strawberries, raspberries, oranges, cranberries, red grapes, black currants, blue plums, onion, and grapefruit, is another way to help reduce the discomfort of osteoarthritis.

Cayenne pepper (capsaicin) cream can ease a painful joint. Natural anti-inflammatories include feverfew, turmeric (500 milligrams twice a day), white willow, yucca, bromelain (500 milligrams twice a day), omega-3 fatty acids (1 tablespoon of flaxseed oil), and quercetin. Exercise has also been shown to be very beneficial in reducing joint swelling, pain, and stiffness. Glucosamine sulfate (1,500 milligrams a day) may actually stimulate joint repair.

Chinese Patent Formulas
Bao Zhen Gao
Du Huo Ji Sheng Wan
Zhui Feng Huo Xue Pian

Herbs
Alfalfa
Black cohosh*
Burdock*
Cayenne pepper*
Chaparral*
Devil's claw*
Dong quai (Dang gui)
Feverfew
Horsetail
Juniper
Licorice
Mustard
Poke
Turmeric*
White willow*
Yucca*

Supplements
Boron
Bromelain*
Cetyl myristoleate*
Copper
DMSO
Glucosamine sulfate*
Methylsulfonylmethane
Niacinamide
Omega-3 fatty acids*
Phenylalanine*
Quercetin
S-adenosylmethionine*
Shark cartilage
Vitamin E

▶ OSTEOPOROSIS

Osteoporosis is a disorder in which the bones become increasingly porous, brittle, and subject to fracture, owing to loss of calcium and other mineral components. It is very common in postmenopausal women between the ages of 50 and 75 because of a natural decrease in estrogen production. Other causes of osteoporosis include overactive thyroid, diabetes, use of corticosteroid drugs or heparin (a blood thinner), tobacco use, immobilization, kidney and liver disease, Crohn's disease, malabsorption syndrome, and rheumatoid arthritis. General lifestyle factors associated with osteoporosis include lack of exercise, nutritional deficiencies, caffeine use, and a high-salt or high-protein diet.

People who have osteoporosis generally remain symptom-free until fracture occurs. Fractures mainly occur in the wrists, hips, and spine. To help prevent osteoporosis, it is important to take a good multivitamin/mineral supplement. Women in their twenties and thirties should take calcium (1,200 milligrams a day) and magnesium (600 milligrams a day) to prevent osteoporosis later in life. (See "Reducing Your Risk of Osteoporosis" on page 126.)

As important as these supplements are, however, studies show that calcium supplementation is not enough and that weight-bearing exercises

good multivitamin/mineral supplement that includes all the B vitamins is recommended because B vitamins affect mood. (Do not take B vitamins separately unless advised to do so by a health care provider, since a high dose of one B vitamin can deplete another.) Eating four small protein meals throughout the day can be calming to the nerves, since people tend to burn more protein during stressful times. A healthy diet high in fresh fruits and vegetables and low in saturated fat can also be helpful during stressful periods. Avoid stimulants such as alcohol, tobacco, and caffeine, which can add more stress to the body.

Exercise is recommended to help the body deal with stressful events. (See "Managing Stress" on pages 18–19.) Herbs that have a calming effect on the body include chamomile, hops, lavender, passionflower, and valerian. (See "Relief for Stress—and Premature Gray Hair" on page 501.)

Herbs
Asian ginseng*
Chamomile*
Hops*
Kava kava+
Lavender*
Passionflower*
Siberian ginseng*
Valerian*

Supplements
B vitamins
Isoleucine
Leucine
Phosphatidylserine
Tyrosine
Valine

▶ STROKE

A stroke is a blockage of or hemorrhage in a blood vessel leading to the brain that causes an inadequate oxygen supply and often long-term impairment of sensation and movement. Symptoms can include a severe headache, dizziness, confusion, difficulty swallowing, or loss of functioning of part of the body. If the brain does not get enough oxygen, parts of the brain may die, causing paralysis, speech problems, numbness, difficulty speaking, blindness, and loss of body functions.

Most strokes are due to hardening of the arteries and high blood pressure. Other health conditions that can increase stroke risk include high cholesterol levels, diabetes, smoking, blood clots in the legs, and heart disease.

Eating a diet high in fruits and vegetables, reducing saturated fat, and taking omega-3 fatty acids and vitamin E can help you reduce your risk for stroke, as can participating in daily exercise. (See "Eating to Cut Your Risk of Stroke" on page 148.) Elevated homocysteine levels have been shown to be a risk factor for developing stroke, heart disease, and other vascular diseases, so folic acid and vitamins B_6 and B_{12} can be taken to lower one's risk of having a stroke. Folic acid and vitamins B_6 and B_{12} have been shown to reduce the incidence of coronary heart disease in women.

If you suspect that you are having a stroke, seek emergency treatment to prevent permanent damage to the blood vessels. Ginkgo has been shown to improve blood circulation to the brain and limbs. Omega-3 fatty acids such as flaxseed oil (1 tablespoon per day) can decrease inflammation and improve circulation.

Chinese Patent Formula
Ren Shen Zai Zao Wan*

Herbs
Ginkgo*
Hawthorn*

Supplements
Coenzyme Q_{10}*
Folic acid*
Magnesium*

*preferred and can be used in combination

Omega-3 fatty acids*
Potassium
Vitamin B$_6$*
Vitamin B$_{12}$
Vitamin E*

▶ STY

A sty, or hordeolum, is an abscess caused by a bacterial infection (usually a staphylococcal infection) of the glands on the edge of the eyelid. A sty can be external, on the eyelid, or internal, involving one of the small glands in the lid that help provide lubrication.

An external sty usually begins with pain, redness, and tenderness of the lid margin. You may have tearing, light sensitivity, and the feeling that a foreign body is in your eye. The abscess generally ruptures on its own, with a discharge of pus. An internal sty is more severe. The pain, redness, and swelling are more localized, spontaneous rupture is rare, and recurrence is common. A topical application of warm witch hazel (applied to the area with a washcloth for 20 minutes three times a day) may draw out an internal or external sty. (Do not use a witch hazel tincture, because the alcohol can burn the eye.) A warm eyebright tea bag or black tea bag held on the infected area can help reduce the redness and inflammation associated with either type of sty. See a health care provider if the infection does not resolve within a couple of days.

Herbs
Echinacea*
Eyebright*
Goldenseal*
Witch hazel

Homeopathic Remedies
Apis mellifica
Graphites
Pulsatilla

Eating to Cut Your Risk of Stroke

Can eating fish, fruits, and vegetables lower your risk of stroke? The evidence suggests that it can. One study of African-American and white women and men aged 45 to 74 showed that those who ate fish more than once a week had fewer strokes than those who didn't eat fish. Another study of 832 men aged 45 to 65, conducted over 20 years and reported in 1995, showed that the risk of stroke lessened with increases in daily servings of fruits and vegetables.

▶ SUNBURN

Sunburn is inflammation of the skin caused by overexposure to the sun or a sunlamp, causing blisters, swelling, and pain. The only way to prevent sunburn and skin cancer is to stay out of the sun. Regardless of the time of year, always wear a hat when outdoors, because sunburn can occur year-round. Sunscreens do not protect you from getting skin cancer. Studies are showing that even though people are using sunscreens, skin cancer rates are increasing. This is because many people are staying in the sun for longer periods of time because they feel that they are protected by sunscreens. This is not true, although it is still advisable to wear sunscreen to avoid sunburn. If you are outdoors for long periods of time, wear sunscreen, keep your skin covered, and drink plenty of water to stay hydrated.

Supplemental vitamins C and E have been shown to protect against getting sunburn. To relieve the burning and itching associated with sunburn, use 100 percent aloe vera juice. A calendula, comfrey, and plantain salve also can be very soothing and healing for sunburn. An oatmeal bath can help with the itching and pain; to prepare a bath, place a cup of oatmeal in cheesecloth and hang the cheesecloth in the warm running water. You also can add powdered milk or lavender oil for an added soothing effect.

Herbs
Aloe vera*
Calendula
Comfrey
Lavender
Plantain

Homeopathic Remedies
Belladonna
Bufo
Cantharis
Ferrum phosphoricum

Supplements
Vitamin C*
Vitamin E*

▶ SURGERY, RECOVERY FROM

Any type of surgery places demands on your body. Nutrients can be used to help speed recovery and reduce inflammation and scarring. Taking supplements of bromelain (500 milligrams twice a day), quercetin (500 milligrams twice a day), and omega-3 fatty acids (1 tablespoon a day of flaxseed oil) for 1 month before elective surgery can help reduce inflammation after the operation. Supplements that promote tissue healing and thus should be included in a good multivitamin/mineral supplement include zinc, vitamin A, beta-carotene, and copper. Taking extra vitamin C (3,000 milligrams a day) and vitamin E (400 international units a day) can help reduce

scarring, as can taking the herb gotu kola. A diet high in fruits and vegetables and low in saturated fat can improve overall healing. After surgery, eat four small protein meals a day, because extra protein is needed in wound repair and healing.

Herb
Gotu kola*

Supplements
Beta-carotene
Bromelain*
Copper
Glutamine
Isoleucine
Leucine
Methionine
Omega-3 fatty acids*
Quercetin*
Valine
Vitamin A*
Vitamin B$_5$ (Pantothenic acid)
Vitamin C*
Vitamin E*
Zinc*

▶ SYSTEMIC LUPUS ERYTHEMATOSUS

See Lupus

▶ TARDIVE DYSKINESIA

Tardive dyskinesia is nerve damage that results in involuntary repetitive movements. Any muscle of the body can be affected, but the movements commonly occur in the face, mouth, or neck. Dyskinesia often develops in people who take long-term courses of antipsychotic medications as a result of up-regulation of dopamine receptors. Therefore, antipsychotic drugs should be discontinued if there are signs of tardive dyskinesia, but not without the supervision of a health care

+use supported by Commission E (p. 160)

provider. Antipsychotic drugs should be discontinued slowly to prevent severe side effects.

Vitamin E at a dose of 800 international units a day has been shown to improve the symptoms of patients suffering from drug-induced tardive dyskinesia. A good multivitamin/mineral supplement is also recommended. Choline and lecithin also can be helpful in reducing the symptoms associated with this condition.

Supplements
- Choline*
- Lecithin*
- Manganese*
- Vitamin E*

▶ TEETHING

Teething is the period during which an infant's teeth begin to erupt through the gums, generally at 5 to 6 months of age. Symptoms of teething include dribbling, chewing on fingers and objects, red and swollen gums, irritability, crying, clinging behavior, sleep disturbance, and lack of appetite. The child also may be more susceptible to fever, earache, upper-respiratory infection, diarrhea, and coughs. (See "Soothing Sara's Teething Pains" on page 390.)

Herbs can be used in teas, baths, glycerites, and tinctures, but consult your physician before administering herbs to children. To help decrease inflammation and numb the gums, saturate a washcloth with an herbal combination, put it in the freezer, then place it on the sore spots in the infant's mouth.

Herbs
- Catnip*
- Chamomile*
- Echinacea*
- Lemon balm*
- Licorice
- White willow

Homeopathic Remedies
- Belladonna
- Calcarea carbonica
- Calcarea phosphorica
- Chamomilla*
- Silicea

▶ THRUSH

Thrush, also known as oral candidiasis, is a fungal infection of the mouth that appears as creamy white patches on the tongue and inner cheeks. It is common in people with depleted immune systems, as in those with AIDS, or in people who are receiving long-term antibiotics, corticosteroids, or cancer medications. Rinsing the mouth with a mixture of ½ cup water and ¼ cup hydrogen peroxide can help clear the infection. Swish the mixture in your mouth three or four times and spit it out (do not swallow it). Since fungus tends to feed on sugar, it is beneficial to eliminate all sugar from the diet. Antifungal herbs include pau d'arco, garlic (three raw cloves a day), and chamomile (drink three cups of tea a day). Thrush also may be associated with intestinal and vaginal candidiasis.

Herbs
- Chamomile*
- Garlic*
- Pau d'arco

Homeopathic Remedies
- Borax
- Chamomilla
- Hydrastis
- Mercurius
- Sulphur

▶ TINNITUS

Tinnitus is the sensation of ringing, buzzing, hissing, roaring, or clicking in the ears. The sound may be intermittent, continuous, or pulsating and be heard in one ear or both. It can be due to an ear infection, a foreign body in the ear, earwax, long-term aspirin use, certain diuretics, heart medications, high blood pressure, Ménière's disease, anemia, underactive thyroid, or head trauma.

Ginkgo (40 milligrams three times a day) has been shown to be effective in treating tinnitus. If you have tinnitus, eat a healthy diet and avoid alcohol and caffeinated beverages, which can make the symptoms worse. A good multivitamin/mineral supplement is also recommended. Craniosacral therapy and biofeedback have been effective in treating tinnitus. See a health care provider to get an accurate diagnosis before using any treatment for tinnitus.

Chinese Patent Formulas
Ba Xian Chang Shou Wan

Er Ming Zuo Ci Wan

Herb
Ginkgo*

Supplements
Calcium

Magnesium

Omega-3 fatty acids*

Vitamin B$_{12}$*

Zinc*

▶ TOOTHACHE

Toothache pain occurs in or around a tooth, usually as a result of a cavity, a gum infection, improper flossing, or an abscess. Foods that may contribute to gum disease, periodontal disease, and cavities include sugar and refined carbohydrates (white flour). A diet high in vegetables, complex carbohydrates, and protein is recommended.

Wintergreen or clove oil can be applied to the sore area to numb the pain. See a dentist if a toothache lasts more than 1 day. The herbs below can reduce the inflammation and support the immune system; however, herbs are not a substitute for proper dental care. To prevent toothache and tooth decay, have your teeth cleaned every 6 months. Also, brush and floss after every meal.

See also Gum Disease; Periodontal Disease

Chinese Patent Formula
Niu Huang Jie Du Pian*

Herbs
Calendula*

Catnip*

Echinacea*

Garlic*

Ginger

Licorice*

Marjoram

Mint

White willow*

▶ ULCERATIVE COLITIS

Ulcerative colitis is a chronic inflammatory and ulcerative disease of the colon, characterized most often by bloody diarrhea. Symptoms include alternating spells of bloody diarrhea and constipation that vary in intensity and duration, abdominal cramps, fever, and weight loss. People with this condition may have 10 to 20 bowel movements in one day.

Ulcerative colitis generally occurs in women between the ages of 15 and 35, and Jewish women have a three to six times higher incidence of the disease compared to other ethnic groups. Possible causes include infection from viruses, candida, or bacteria; parasites; a depressed immune system; or food allergies. Ulcerative colitis (both in first onset and in subsequent flare-ups) generally occurs after emotional or physical stress.

A diet high in fiber and complex carbohy-

*preferred and can be used in combination

drates may be beneficial in relieving symptoms associated with ulcerative colitis. Many people with ulcerative colitis are deficient in calcium, folic acid, iron, magnesium, potassium, vitamins A, C, and E, and zinc; therefore, a good multivitamin/mineral supplement is recommended. An elimination diet can help relieve the symptoms caused by allergies. (See "How to Tell If You Have Food Allergies" on page 26.)

Glutamine (1,000 milligrams twice a day) is an amino acid that can help heal the intestinal lining. Chamomile or peppermint tea (three cups a day) can help relieve the cramps associated with ulcerative colitis. Digestive herbs such as dandelion, gentian, peppermint, or wormwood can help relieve constipation, gas, and bloating. Any sign of blood in the stool is reason to see a doctor immediately, because this can be a sign of cancer.

Herbs
Chamomile*
Dandelion
Echinacea
Gentian*
Goldenseal
Licorice
Mint*
Wormwood*
Yellow dock*

Supplements
Calcium*
DHEA
Digestive enzymes
Folic acid*
Glutamine*
Iron
Magnesium*
Omega-6 fatty acids
Potassium
Quercetin*
Vitamin A*
Vitamin C*
Vitamin E*
Zinc*

▶ UNDERACTIVE THYROID (HYPOTHYROIDISM)

Hypothyroidism is caused by insufficient production of thyroid hormone by the body. Symptoms include fatigue, weight gain, dry hair and skin, loss of concentration, constipation, slow heart rate, heavy menstrual periods, numbness and coldness in the hands and feet, and anemia. Men are very unlikely to have hypothyroidism.

Women who have problems becoming pregnant may want to have their thyroid levels checked, because low levels of thyroid hormones can affect estrogen and progesterone levels, thus causing infertility. Many women have subclinical underactive thyroid, which means that low levels of thyroid hormone do not show up on thyroid tests yet they may have many of the symptoms. The basal body temperature test was discovered by Rhoda Barnes, M.D. Dr. Barnes found that many patients who had the symptoms of underactive thyroid had normal thyroid levels on the lab test. She found that the basal body temperature was a better indicator than the thyroid lab test because the lab test is not sensitive enough to pick up subclinical underactive thyroid. You can test for subclinical underactive thyroid yourself, at home. (See "How to Check for Underactive Thyroid" on page 154.)

Supplements that help stimulate the thyroid include kelp, poke, iodine, and tyrosine. A good multivitamin/mineral supplement is also recommended.

Herbs
Black walnut
Kelp*
Poke*
Siberian ginseng

Supplements

- Iodine*
- Tyrosine
- Vitamin A*
- Vitamin B$_2$ (Riboflavin)
- Vitamin B$_3$ (Niacin)
- Zinc*

▶ UTERINE CRAMPS

See Menstrual Cramps

▶ VAGINITIS

Vaginitis is an inflammation of the vagina. Symptoms include vaginal itching and burning, odor, increased frequency of urination, pain on urination, and a white or yellow discharge. Vaginitis can be caused by candida, protozoa (trichomonas), bacteria (gardnerella), parasites (chlamydia), gonorrhea, or atrophy (seen in postmenopausal women because of thinning of the vaginal wall). The most common cause is candida. Factors that predispose a woman to candidiasis include the use of antibiotics, birth control pills, or corticosteroid drugs; a diet high in sugar; or diabetes. Vaginitis can be sexually transmitted, so it is important to get an accurate diagnosis from a health care provider for proper treatment.

If you have vaginitis, eat a diet rich in vegetables, whole grains, and proteins and avoid all sugar, refined carbohydrates, dairy products, and alcohol. Wearing 100 percent cotton underwear, bleached to kill the bacteria and yeast at every washing, is recommended. Eating natural low-fat yogurt can help restore the acidophilus (good bacteria) in the colon and vagina. If you take antibiotics, acidophilus supplementation is recommended to help avoid candida-type infection.

Chinese Patent Formulas

- Qian Jin Zhi Dai Wan
- Yu Dai Wan

Herbs

- Echinacea
- Garlic*
- Goldenseal*
- Oregon grape
- Pau d'arco*
- Tea tree

Homeopathic Remedies

- Borax
- Calcarea carbonica
- Graphites
- Kreosotum
- Nitricum acidum
- Pulsatilla
- Sepia

Supplements

- Beta-carotene
- Vitamin A
- Vitamin C*

▶ VARICOSE VEINS

Varicose veins are abnormally enlarged, permanently distended, dilated veins that often occur in the calves and lower legs. Symptoms include aching/burning pain, swelling, and leg fatigue that is often relieved by elevating the leg or wearing support hose. Symptoms may worsen during the menstrual period or with pregnancy. Other health conditions associated with varicose veins include obesity, standing or sitting for long periods of time, constipation, and hemorrhoids.

Eating a high-fiber diet, exercising regularly, not standing for long periods, and maintaining your ideal weight can help reduce the symptoms of varicose veins. Foods high in bioflavonoids protect, strengthen, and stabilize collagen, which is a component of connective tissue and blood vessels; therefore, bioflavonoids may help prevent

+use supported by Commission E (p. 160)

How to Check for Underactive Thyroid

One of the best ways to check thyroid function is to monitor your basal body temperature. Basal body temperature reflects the thyroid gland's impact on your metabolic rate. A basal body temperature that is consistently below 97.6 degrees over a 5-day period may indicate low thyroid function.

Here's how to measure your basal body temperature.

1. Shake down an oral glass thermometer to below 95 degrees. Put it beside your bed before you go to sleep.

2. When you awaken, before you get out of bed, place the thermometer under your armpit or in your mouth. Remain still for 10 minutes. The less you move, the more accurate the reading.

3. Record your temperature, and the date. For ovulating women, it's best if the test is started on the first day of the menstrual cycle. If you don't know where you are in your cycle, record your basal body temperature on a separate piece of paper until you begin menses. Then, on the first day of menstruation, start numbering again, beginning with Day 1.

4. Record your temperature for 5 days. Then, show your chart to your naturopathic physician, who can use it to help determine if you suffer from low thyroid function.

varicose veins. Eat ½ to 1 cup a day of foods high in bioflavonoids, such as blueberries, grapefruit, oranges, cranberries, red grapes, raspberries, black currants, and plums. (See "Homeopathy-Based Treatment for Varicose Veins" on page 410.) Herbs that have been shown to be beneficial include bilberry, ginkgo, gotu kola, horse chestnut, and witch hazel. Omega-3 fatty acids (1 tablespoon a day of flaxseed oil) can help improve circulation and decrease the inflammation. A good multivitamin/mineral supplement is also recommended.

Herbs
Bilberry*
Burdock
Comfrey
Ginkgo*
Gotu kola*
Horse chestnut*
Witch hazel*

Homeopathic Remedies
Arnica montana
Calcarea carbonica
Hamamelis
Lachesis
Pulsatilla

Supplements
Bromelain*
Omega-3 fatty acids*
Vitamin C*
Vitamin E*

▶ VIRAL INFECTION

There are several hundred different viruses that may infect humans. They are spread mainly by respiratory secretions and through the gastrointestinal tract. Common diseases caused by viruses include herpes simplex, influenza, mumps, Epstein-Barr, measles, hepatitis, and warts. The herbs and supplements listed below have antiviral properties.

Herbs
Echinacea*
Lemon balm
Licorice*

Supplements
Lysine*
Vitamin A*
Vitamin C*
Zinc*

▶ VITILIGO

Vitiligo is a skin condition of unknown origin that causes loss of pigmentation. It can range from affecting only one or two areas to affecting the skin of the whole body. Vitiligo has been associated with diabetes, Addison's disease, deficient stomach acid, pernicious anemia, and thyroid disorders. One study shows that folic acid and vitamin B_{12} supplementation combined with sun exposure can induce repigmentation in people with vitiligo. Other substances that are often deficient in people with vitiligo include digestive enzymes, para-aminobenzoic acid, and phenylalanine.

Supplements
Digestive enzymes*
Folic acid*
Para-aminobenzoic acid*
Phenylalanine
Vitamin B_{12}*
Vitamin C

▶ WHIPLASH

Whiplash is pain in the neck as a result of sudden, violent movements of the neck, such as often occur during automobile accidents. A neck brace and physical therapy can be beneficial for re-strengthening the neck muscles. See a health care provider for an accurate diagnosis if you experience pain after a trauma. Phenylalanine supplementation at a dose of 250 milligrams three or four times a day has been shown to be effective in treating chronic pain.

Supplement
Phenylalanine*

▶ WHOOPING COUGH (PERTUSSIS)

Whooping cough is an infectious disease caused by the *Bordetella pertussis* bacteria and characterized by peculiar paroxysms of coughing that end in prolonged whooping breaths. It is transmitted by coughing. Symptoms include sneezing, fatigue, hacking cough, choking spells from the cough, and vomiting. Whooping cough is a serious disease in children under 2 years old because it can cause asphyxia and pneumonia. See a health care provider for an accurate diagnosis. The herbs listed below can be soothing to the throat.

Chinese Patent Formula
Luo Han Guo Chong Ji
Herbs
Elecampane*
Garlic*
Lobelia*
Mullein*
Thyme*

▶ WOUNDS

A wound is an injury that involves division of tissue or rupture of the mucous membrane as a result of either trauma to the body or a surgical incision. Common types include open wounds, penetrating wounds, puncture wounds, stab wounds, and abraded wounds. If the wound is bleeding, cover the area with a clean cloth or bandage and apply firm pressure. If the bleeding does not stop within 5 minutes, seek emergency help as soon as possible. If the wound is not bleeding,

*preferred and can be used in combination

clean the area with hydrogen peroxide and apply a clean bandage.

Common herbs that are used topically in a salve to promote wound healing are calendula, comfrey, plantain, and St. John's wort. If a wound is red, swollen, or painful, see a health care provider, since these symptoms can indicate infection. A good multivitamin/mineral supplement is also recommended to promote healing. Adequate protein is also needed to promote healing, so if you have a wound, you should eat four small protein meals a day that include foods such as chicken, fish, soy, nuts, and seeds.

Herbs

Calendula*
Comfrey*
Echinacea
Fenugreek
Gotu kola*
Juniper
Plantain*
Rhubarb

Rosemary
St. John's wort*
Slippery elm
Stinging nettle
Sweet woodruff
Thyme
Witch hazel
Yarrow

Homeopathic Remedies

Apis mellifica
Hepar sulphuris
Hypericum
Ledum
Silicea

Supplements

Arginine
Bromelain*
Glycine
Histidine
Proline
Vitamin A*
Vitamin C
Vitamin E*
Zinc*

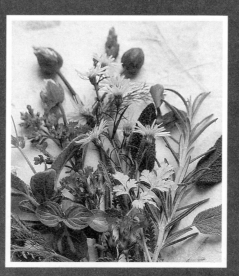

PART 3

HEALING
WITH
HERBS

- Flatulence
- Hot flashes
- Menopausal symptoms
- Menstrual cramps
- Osteoarthritis
- Premenstrual syndrome

▶ ECHINACEA

Botanical Names

Echinacea angustifolia, E. purpurea

Other Names

Black sampson, purple cornflower

Family

Asteraceae

Description

Echinacea is a perennial that grows in open woods, along roadsides, and in fields from Texas to southern Canada. It has sturdy stems covered with tiny, bristly hairs. Its cone-shaped purple flowers bloom from mid- to late summer.

Parts Used

Root, whole herb

Forms Used

Tincture, tea, capsules, tablets, salve

Dosage

Tincture: ½ teaspoon (40 drops or 2.5 milliliters) three times a day. Tea: 1 tablespoon per cup of water; three cups a day. Capsules and tablets: 200 milligrams twice a day. Salve: Use topically on wounds as needed.

Characteristics

Antibacterial, antiviral, blood tonic, vulnerary, hastens tissue renewal

Cautions

Echinacea has been shown to lose its immunity-boosting effects when taken for more than 2 weeks at a time. It may cause allergic reactions in some people. Echinacea should not be taken without consulting a physician if you have an autoimmune disease such as tuberculosis or multiple sclerosis. Echinacea is safe during pregnancy and lactation.

Active Ingredients

Essential oils, resins, flavonoids, mucilage, polysaccharides, alkaloids

Use

- Bacterial infections
- Bladder infections
- Bronchitis
- Canker sores
- Chronic fatigue syndrome
- Colds
- Coughs
- Ear infections
- Fever
- Fibromyalgia
- Herpes simplex
- Immunodeficiency
- Influenza
- Laryngitis
- Lymph node swelling
- Measles and rubella
- Mononucleosis
- Mumps
- Sinusitis
- Sore throat
- Sty
- Teething
- Toothache
- Ulcerative colitis
- Vaginitis
- Viral infection
- Wounds

▶ ELDERBERRY

Botanical Name

Sambucus canadensis

Other Names

American elder, sambucus, sweet elder

Family

Caprifoliaceae

Description

Elder is a shrub that grows in low, damp areas in all parts of the United States. The trees grow 5 to 12 feet tall, with star-shaped flowers that bloom in June and July. The purple-black berries mature in September and October; they are often used to make jellies, pies, and wine.

Parts Used

Flowers, berries

Forms Used

Tincture, tea

Dosage

Tincture: ¼ teaspoon (20 drops or 1.3 milliliters) three times a day. Tea: 1 tablespoon per cup of water; three cups a day.

Characteristics

Antiviral, anti-inflammatory, antiallergenic

Cautions

The roots, stems, leaves, and uncooked berries of elder are poisonous. Long-term use of elderberry can be toxic to the liver.

Active Ingredients

Triterpenes, free fatty acids, fixed oils, flavonoids, tannins, alkaloids

Use

- Colds
- Fever
- Hay fever
- Inflammation
- Influenza
- Laryngitis
- Sinusitis

▶ ELECAMPANE

Botanical Name

Inula helenium

Other Names

Aunee, elf dock, scabwort, velvet dock, wild sunflower

Family

Asteraceae or Compositae

Description

Elecampane is a perennial with toothed leaves that have velvety undersides. It is indigenous to Europe and Asia and is naturalized in the United States.

Part Used

Root

Forms Used

Tincture, tea

Dosage

Tincture: ½ teaspoon (40 drops or 2.5 milliliters) three times a day. Tea: 1 tablespoon per cup of water; three cups a day.

Characteristics

Diuretic, expectorant, antiparasitic, antibacterial, antifungal, expectorant, diaphoretic, tonic

Cautions

Elecampane may cause irritation of the mucous membranes and contact dermatitis in some people.

Active Ingredients

Essential oil, saponins, mucilage, inulin, resin

Use

- Asthma
- Bronchitis
- Candidiasis (intestinal)
- Coughs
- Diarrhea
- Indigestion
- Intestinal infection

- Stomach cramps
- Whooping cough

▶ EUCALYPTUS

Botanical Name

Eucalyptus globulus

Other Names

Blue gum tree, fevertree, Tasmanian blue gum

Family

Myrtaceae

Description

There are more than 500 species of eucalyptus, ranging from 5-foot shrubs to 480-foot trees. The majority are evergreens with thick, dark green, sword-shaped leaves. All types produce an oil with a strong menthol odor. Eucalyptus is native to Australia and Tasmania and is cultivated in southern Europe and the southwestern United States.

Part Used

Leaves

Form Used

Essential oil

Dosage

1 to 5 drops (0.067 to 0.33 milliliter) two or three times a day

Characteristics

Antibacterial, antiseptic, antispasmodic, expectorant, stimulant

Cautions

Eucalyptus oil should be taken internally only in very small doses. It is often an ingredient in cough syrups, sweets, and pastilles; it can also be used as an inhalant to break up sputum in coughs and colds. Large doses of eucalyptus taken internally can cause nausea, vomiting, diarrhea, and muscle spasms. When applied topically, eucalyptus oil should be diluted with water. Eucalyptus can cause an allergic reac-

tion in sensitive individuals. It is contraindicated in individuals with bile duct inflammation or obstruction, gastrointestinal inflammation, or liver disease. It should not be used internally in children under age 1.

Active Ingredients

Volatile oil, sesquiterpenes, polyphenolic acids, flavonoids

Use

- Abscesses
- Asthma
- Bronchitis
- Colds
- Croup
- Joint pain

▶ EVENING PRIMROSE

Botanical Name

Oenothera biennis

Other Names

Tree primrose, sundrop

Family

Onagraceae

Description

Evening primrose is a perennial with alternate, lanceolate leaves and large, yellow, four-petalled flowers. It is native to the United States and grows mainly on sandy soil. It is a common garden plant.

Part Used

Leaves, seeds

Forms Used

Oil, capsules

Dosage

Oil: 1 tablespoon (2 to 6 grams) a day. Capsules: 500 milligrams, three times a day.

Characteristics

Anti-inflammatory, antispasmodic, vasodilator, blood-thinner

Cautions

None known

Active Ingredients

Gamma-linolenic acid (omega-6 fatty acid)

Cautions

Evening primrose is best taken in conjuction with vitamin E to prevent oxidation. Other nutrients that may help evening primrose oil convert to prostaglandin E_1, a fatty acid that possesses its anti-inflammatory, antispasmodic, vasodilator, and blood-thinner effects, include magnesium and vitamins B_6 and C.

Use

- Attention deficit hyperactivity disorder
- Breast tenderness
- Coronary heart disease
- Dandruff
- Diabetes
- Dyspepsia
- Eczema
- Fibrocystic breasts
- High blood pressure
- Menstrual cramps
- Premenstrual syndrome
- Rheumatoid arthritis

▶ EYEBRIGHT

Botanical Name

Euphrasia officinalis

Other Names

Euphrasia, casse-lunette, augentrost

Family

Scrophulariaceae

Description

Eyebright is an annual that grows 2 to 8 inches tall. It has oval leaves and white or purple flowers that are often tinged with yellow spots. Eyebright is found in meadows and grassy areas in England, Europe, and western Asia.

Part Used

Whole herb

Forms Used

Tincture, tea

Dosage

Tincture: ¼ teaspoon (20 drops or 1.3 milliliters) three times a day. Tea: 1 tablespoon per cup of water; four cups a day. For conjunctivitis, use a warm tea bag or dip a washcloth in the tea and place it over the affected eye for 15 minutes three times a day.

Characteristics

Astringent, hastens tissue renewal, liver tonic

Cautions

Make sure eyebright preparations applied to the eye are sterile; unsterile homemade preparations can worsen an eye infection.

Active Ingredients

Tannins, pseudotannin, resin, flavonoids, quercetin, volatile oil

Use

- Conjunctivitis
- Dry eyes
- Hay fever
- Sinusitis
- Sty

▶ FENNEL

Botanical Name

Foeniculum vulgare

Other Names

Fenkel, sweet fennel, wild fennel

Family

Umbelliferae

Description

Fennel is a perennial that is often cultivated as an annual. The feathery leaves are alternately branched on broad stems, and the small yellow flowers bloom from July to October. Fennel is native to the Mediterranean region and is widely cultivated.

Part Used

Whole herb

Forms Used

Seeds, tincture, and tea

Dosage

Seeds: chew 5 to 10 after meals for indigestion or colic. Tincture: ¼ teaspoon (20 drops or 1.3 milliliters) three times a day. Tea: 1 tablespoon per cup of water; three cups a day.

Characteristics

Aromatic, antispasmodic, carminative, diuretic, expectorant, stimulant, anti-inflammatory

Cautions

Fennel may cause allergic reactions in some people.

Active Ingredients

Volatile oils, terpenes, resins, saponins, flavonoids, coumarins

Use

- Bad breath
- Breastfeeding (complications of)
- Colic
- Coughs
- Dyspepsia
- Flatulence
- Hot flashes
- Indigestion
- Insufficient lactation
- Menopausal symptoms
- Stomach cramps

▶ FENUGREEK

Botanical Name

Trigonella foenum-graecum

Other Names

Bird's foot, Greek hayseed

Family

Leguminosae

Description

Fenugreek is an annual with stems and leaves that slightly resemble clover. The oblong, toothed leaves are ¾ to 2 inches long. The flowers, which bloom in midsummer, have curved seed pods and are 2 to 3 inches long. Fenugreek is native to western Asia and the Mediterranean and is cultivated in North America.

Part Used

Seeds

Forms Used

Tincture, tea, defatted seed powder

Dosage

Tincture: ½ teaspoon (40 drops or 2.5 milliliters) three times a day. Tea: 1 tablespoon per cup of water; three cups a day. Defatted seed powder: Mix 50 grams with 8 ounces of water or juice; twice a day with meals. For wounds and boils, dissolve 50 grams of powder in ¼ liter of water and apply topically.

Characteristics

Expectorant, laxative, demulcent, emollient, astringent

Cautions

Fenugreek is generally regarded as safe.

Active Ingredients

Resins, saponins, alkaloids, flavonoids, mucilage

Use

- Boils
- Breastfeeding (complications of)
- Constipation
- Cough
- Diabetes
- Hay fever
- High cholesterol levels
- Low blood sugar
- Wounds

▶ FEVERFEW

Botanical Name

Tanacetum parthenium

Other Names

Featherfew, featherfoil, pyrethrum, wild quinine

Family

Asteraceae or Compositae

Description

Feverfew can be a biennial or a perennial and is a member of the daisy family. The greenish yellow leaves are bitterly scented and about 4 inches long. The numerous flowers are white and daisy-like. Feverfew is native to central and southern Europe and is naturalized in North America.

Parts Used

Whole herb, leaves

Forms Used

Tea, standardized extract

Dosage

Tea: 1 tablespoon per cup of water; three cups a day. Standardized extract: One 100-milligram capsule twice a day (250 micrograms of parthenolides a day).

Characteristics

Digestant, anti-inflammatory, analgesic, tranquilizing, induces menstruation

Cautions

Do not use during pregnancy or lactation. Feverfew may increase the anti-clotting effect of aspirin. Feverfew is not recommended for children under age 5.

Active Ingredients

Essential oil, sesquiterpene lactones, terpenes

Use

- Abdominal pain
- Fever
- Headache
- Joint pain
- Lower-back pain
- Menstrual cramps
- Migraine
- Muscle strain
- Osteoarthritis
- Rheumatoid arthritis

▶ FLAX

Botanical Name

Linum usitatissimum

Other Names

Flaxseed, linseed

Family

Linaceae

Description

Flax has a solitary stem that branches at the top and pale green leaves shaped like spearheads. The light blue flowers bloom from June through August. Flax is cultivated throughout the northwestern United States, Canada, and Europe.

Part Used

Seeds

Forms Used

Oil, seeds

Dosage

Oil or seeds: 1 to 2 tablespoons a day

Characteristics

Demulcent, laxative, emollient

Cautions

The immature seed pods of flax are toxic, as is boiled flaxseed oil. Keep the oil refrigerated to prevent rancidity, and never heat it. Taking other drugs with flaxseed may delay their absorption. Do not use if you have intestinal colic. Flaxseed is a natural blood-thinner and may interact with drugs such as Coumadin.

Active Ingredients

Essential oil, resin, acetic acid, glucoside lina-marin

Use

- Asthma
- Constipation
- Rheumatoid arthritis

▶ GARLIC

Botanical Name

Allium sativum

Other Names

Allium, nectar of the gods, poor-man's treacle, stinking rose

Family

Liliaceae

Description

Garlic is a member of the onion family, with a compound bulb composed of 4 to 15 cloves. The flowers, which bloom in spring and summer, are white to pink. Garlic is cultivated worldwide.

Part Used

Bulbs

Forms Used

Tincture, cloves, oil, standardized extract

Dosage

Tincture: 1 teaspoon (80 drops or 5 milliliters) three times a day. Cloves: Eat two or three a day. Oil: Apply 5 drops (0.33 milliliter) topically for earache, ear infection, or fungal infection on the skin twice a day. Standardized extract: 400 milligrams (containing 5,000 micrograms of al-licin), two to three capsules a day.

Characteristics

Antibacterial, antifungal, anti-yeast, antipara-sitic, hypocholesterolemic, anti-atheroscle-rotic, anticancer, expectorant

Cautions

Placing garlic directly on the skin may cause blisters and a burning sensation. Large doses may interact with the blood-thinner Coumadin.

Active Ingredients

Volatile oil, alliin, allicin, terpenes, resin, flavonoids

Use

- Abscesses
- Asthma
- Bacterial infections
- Bladder infection
- Bronchitis
- Cancer
- Candidiasis (intestinal)
- Colds
- Coronary heart disease
- Coughs
- Diabetes
- Earache
- Ear infections
- Fibromyalgia
- Fungal infections
- Hepatitis
- High blood pressure
- High blood sugar
- High cholesterol levels
- HIV infection and AIDS
- Immunodeficiency
- Influenza
- Intermittent claudication
- Intestinal infection
- Laryngitis
- Low blood sugar
- Measles and rubella
- Mononucleosis
- Mumps
- Parasitic infection
- Sinusitis

- Sore throat
- Stomach cancer
- Thrush
- Toothache
- Vaginitis
- Whooping cough

▶ GENTIAN

Botanical Name

Gentiana lutea

Other Names

Stemless gentian, yellow gentian

Family

Gentianaceae

Description

Gentian is a perennial with a thick root 1 to 2 feet long. When fresh, the root is yellow inside, brown outside, and very bitter. The large yellow flowers bloom from July to August. Gentian is native to the mountains of Europe and is cultivated in the northwestern United States.

Part Used

Root

Form Used

Tincture

Dosage

¼ teaspoon (20 drops or 1.3 milliliters) 10 to 20 minutes before meals three times a day

Characteristics

Digestant, anti-inflammatory, tonic, choleretic

Cautions

Do not use gentian during pregnancy because it may cause nausea and vomiting. Do not use if you have a gastric or duodenal ulcer or heartburn because it can increase the production of stomach acid. Gentian can cause allergic reactions in sensitive people.

Active Ingredients

Volatile oil, bitter compounds, alkaloids, flavonoids

Use

- Anorexia nervosa
- Appetite (loss of)
- Bad breath
- Constipation
- Diarrhea
- Dysentery
- Dyspepsia
- Flatulence
- Food poisoning
- Gout
- Hangover
- Indigestion
- Intestinal atrophy
- Iron-deficiency anemia
- Jaundice
- Menstrual cramps
- Nausea
- Parasitic infection
- Ulcerative colitis

▶ GINGER

Botanical Name

Zingiber officinale

Other Names

Canada snake root, Indian ginger

Family

Zingibcraceae

Description

Ginger is a tropical perennial that rarely flowers in cultivation. It is native to southeast Asia and is cultivated everywhere in the tropics.

Part Used

Root

Forms Used

Tincture, tea, capsules

Dosage

Tincture: ½ teaspoon (40 drops or 2.5 milli-liters) three times a day. Tea: 1 tablespoon per cup of water; three cups a day. Capsules: 300 milligrams twice a day.

Characteristics

Stimulant, diaphoretic, carminative, anti-inflammatory, analgesic, eases gripping intestinal pain

Cautions

Do not use if you have gallstones. The doses listed above are considered safe for pregnancy.

Active Ingredients

Essential oil, terpenes, lecithin, saturated fatty acids

Use

- Bile flow obstruction
- Bronchitis
- Colds
- Coronary heart disease
- Coughs
- Dyspepsia
- Fibromyalgia
- Flatulence
- Headache
- High cholesterol levels
- Influenza
- Laryngitis
- Low blood sugar
- Measles and rubella
- Mononucleosis
- Morning sickness
- Motion sickness
- Mumps
- Nausea
- Pregnancy complications
- Radiation exposure
- Sore throat
- Stomach cancer
- Stomach cramps
- Toothache
- Vomiting

▶ GINKGO

Botanical Name

Ginkgo biloba

Other Name

Maidenhair tree

Family

Ginkgoaceae

Description

Ginkgo, a tree with fan-shaped leaves, is indigenous to China and Japan and is cultivated worldwide.

Part Used

Leaves

Forms Used

Tincture, standardized extract

Dosage

Tincture: ¼ teaspoon (20 drops or 1.3 milli-liters) three times a day. Standardized extract: One 40- to 80-milligram capsule (containing 24 percent glycosides and 6 percent lactones) three times a day.

Characteristics

Digestant, vasodilator, circulatory stimulant, antioxidant, bronchodilator

Cautions

Ginkgo may cause allergic reactions in sensitive people. Signs of overdose are irritability, restlessness, headache, diarrhea, and vomiting. Gingko may increase the effects of anti-clotting drugs such as Coumadin.

Active Ingredients

Volatile oil, terpenes, tannins, flavonoids, lignans, glycosides

Use

- Aging
- Alzheimer's disease
- Asthma
- Bronchitis
- Congestive heart failure
- Coronary heart disease
- Depression
- Diabetes
- Diabetic neuropathy
- Emphysema
- Headache
- Impotence
- Intermittent claudication
- Leg cramps
- Leg ulcers
- Macular degeneration
- Multiple sclerosis
- Parkinson's disease
- Poor circulation
- Poor concentration/memory
- Raynaud's disease
- Schizophrenia
- Seizures
- Stroke
- Tinnitus
- Varicose veins

▶ GOLDENROD

Botanical Name

Solidago virgaurea

Other Names

Aaron's rod, goldruthe, woundwort

Family

Asteraceae or Compositae

Description

Goldenrod is native to North America. It is a perennial with woody stems, and its clusters of yellow flowers bloom in August and September.

Part Used

Whole herb

Form Used

Tea

Dosage

1 tablespoon per cup of water; three cups a day

Characteristics

Astringent, carminative, diuretic, diaphoretic, anti-inflammatory, antiseptic

Cautions

Goldenrod pollen may cause allergic reactions in some people.

Active Ingredients

Saponins, phenolic glucosides, rutin, quercetin, tannins, phenolic acids, polysaccharides

Use

- Bladder infection
- Flatulence
- Kidney stones

▶ GOLDENSEAL

Botanical Name

Hydrastis canadensis

Other Names

Ground raspberry, turmeric root, yellow puccoon

Family

Ranunculaceae

Description

Goldenseal is a perennial with a straight, hairy stem and heart-shaped leaves. The rhizome is covered with yellow-brown bark and is bright yellow on the inside. The herb is native to North America and grows in moist, rich woodlands and damp meadows.

Part Used

Root

Forms Used

Tincture, capsules, tablets, salve

Dosage

Tincture: ½ teaspoon (40 drops or 2.5 milliliters) three times a day for a maximum of 2 weeks. Capsules and tablets: 100 milligrams three times a day for a maximum of 2 weeks. Salve: Apply topically for skin infections as needed.

Characteristics

Antibacterial, antiviral, mild sedative, digestant, antiseptic, hastens tissue renewal, diuretic, astringent, liver tonic, anti-inflammatory

Cautions

Do not use during pregnancy or lactation. Goldenseal may damage normal organisms in the gastrointestinal and genitourinary tracts. High doses may interfere with B vitamin metabolism. Goldenseal should not be used for longer than 2 weeks.

Active Ingredients

Tannin, gallic acid, alkaloids, berberine, hydrastine, canadine, resin, volatile oil

Use

- Abscesses
- Bacterial infections
- Bladder infections
- Boils
- Bronchitis
- Candidiasis (intestinal)
- Chronic fatigue syndrome
- Colds
- Contact dermatitis
- Coughs
- Cuts and scrapes
- Diarrhea
- Dysentery
- Ear infection
- Fever
- Fibromyalgia
- Food poisoning
- Gastritis
- HIV infection and AIDS
- Indigestion
- Influenza
- Measles and rubella
- Mononucleosis
- Parasitic infection
- Peptic ulcer
- Sinusitis
- Sore throat
- Sty
- Ulcerative colitis
- Vaginitis

▶ GOTU KOLA

Botanical Name

Centella asiatica

Other Names

Centella, Indian pennywort, Indian water navelwort

Family

Umbelliferae

Description

Gotu kola is an herbaceous perennial that grows in damp, swampy areas of India, China, Indonesia, Australia, the South Pacific, and southern and central Africa. It is a common Ayurvedic herb.

Parts Used

Whole herb, leaves

Forms Used

Tincture, tea, capsules

Dosage

Tincture: ½ teaspoon (40 drops or 2.5 milliliters) three times a day. Tea: 1 tablespoon per cup of water; three cups a day. Capsules: 100 milligrams a day.

Characteristics

Sedative, tonic, digestant, hastens tissue renewal, nervine, diuretic

Cautions

Do not use during pregnancy or lactation. Very large doses of gotu kola may cause stupor, headache, and coma.

Active Ingredients

Volatile oil, triterpenes, asiatic acid, madecassic acid, saponins, pectin, flavonoids, resins

Use

- Aging
- Alzheimer's disease
- Bruises
- Burns
- Depression
- Enlarged scars
- Fever
- Leg cramps
- Leg ulcers
- Poor concentration/memory
- Surgery (recovery from)
- Varicose veins
- Venous insufficiency
- Wounds

▶ GREEN TEA

Botanical Name

Camellia sinensis

Other Names

Chinese tea, gunpowder

Family

Theaceade

Description

Green tea is a bitter, aromatic beverage prepared by infusing leaves in boiling water. Cultivated mainly in China, India, and Japan, it is derived from the same plant as black tea; the main difference is that green tea is produced by lightly steaming freshly cut leaves, whereas black tea leaves are allowed to oxidize.

Part Used

Leaves

Forms Used

Tea, capsules, standardized extract

Dosage

Tea: 1 tablespoon per cup of tea; 10 cups a day as cancer treatment, 3 cups as preventive. Capsules and standardized extract: 600 to 1,250 milligrams (containing 80 percent polyphenol and 55 percent epigallocatechin) a day as cancer treatment.

Characteristics

Antioxidant, anticancer, antineoplastic

Cautions

Avoid drinking green tea when boiling hot—extremely hot beverages can cause oral cancer. Green tea contains 3 percent caffeine and may have a stimulating effect on some people, causing nervousness, anxiety, insomnia, and irritability.

Active Ingredients

Catechin, epicatechin, epicatechin gallate, epigallocatechin gallate, proanthocyanidins

Use

- Breast cancer
- Colorectal cancer
- Gum disease
- High blood pressure
- High cholesterol levels
- HIV infection and AIDS
- Lung cancer
- Periodontal disease
- Radiation exposure
- Skin cancer
- Stomach cancer

- Indigestion
- Menstrual periods (lack of)

▶ SAGE

Botanical Name

Salvia officinalis

Other Names

Golden sage, wild sage

Family

Labiatae

Description

Sage is a perennial shrub with square woody stems that are covered with down. The long-stalked leaves are grayish green and hairy with round-toothed margins. Sage is native to the northern Mediterranean coast and is widely cultivated.

Part Used

Leaves

Forms Used

Tincture, tea

Dosage

Tincture: ½ teaspoon (40 drops or 2.5 milliliters) three times a day. Tea: 1 tablespoon per cup of water; three cups a day.

Characteristics

Tonic, antiseptic, astringent, expectorant, antispasmodic, stimulant, immunostimulant, diaphoretic, anti-inflammatory

Cautions

Sage should be used with caution in pregnant or lactating women because it can dry up the breast milk.

Active Ingredients

Volatile oil, terpenes, tannins, phenolic acids, flavonoids

Use

- Bruises
- Colds

- Coughs
- Cuts and scrapes
- Dyspepsia
- Flatulence
- Gum disease
- Hot flashes
- Laryngitis
- Menopausal symptoms
- Menstrual bleeding (excessive)
- Mouth irritation
- Periodontal disease
- Sinusitis
- Sore throat

▶ ST. JOHN'S WORT

Botanical Name

Hypericum perforatum

Other Names

Goatweed, hypericum, klamath weed

Family

Hypericuceae

Description

St. John's wort is a perennial that grows abundantly in woods and meadows in Europe and the United States. The stems are woody, upright, and slender. The leaves are opposite and have transparent holes or black spots on the undersurface. The plant's five-petaled yellow flowers bloom in July and August.

Part Used

Flowering tops

Forms Used

Tincture, tea, standardized extract, salve

Dosage

Tincture: ½ teaspoon (40 drops or 2.5 milliters) three times a day. For ear infection, apply tincture of equal parts St. John's wort and mullein oil, 5 drops (0.33 milliliter) in both ears. Tea: 1 tablespoon per cup of water; three cups a day.

Standardized extract: One 300-milligram capsule (0.3 percent hypericin) three times a day. Salve: Apply topically as needed to insect bites, wounds, cuts and scrapes.

Characteristics

Antibacterial, astringent, sedative, anti-inflammatory

Cautions

St. John's wort should not be used by individuals taking antidepressants because it may interact with selective serotonin reuptake inhibitor drugs, such as Prozac. St. John's wort should not be taken during pregnancy or lactation. Foods containing tyramine should be avoided while taking MAO (monoamine oxidase) inhibitor–type drugs and while taking St. John's wort. These foods include cheese, beer, red wine, herring, beef or chicken liver, fava beans, caffeine, and chocolate. St. John's wort can induce photosensitivity in some individuals.

Active Ingredients

Essential oil, hypericins, flavonoids, epicatechin

Use

- Anxiety attacks
- Bruises
- Burns
- Cuts and scrapes
- Depression
- Dyspepsia
- Ear infection
- Insect bites
- Muscle strain
- Shingles
- Wounds

▶ SAW PALMETTO

Botanical Name

Serenoa repens

Other Names

Hook, sabal

Family

Palmae

Description

Saw palmetto is a shrub with a horizontal, aboveground creeping stem. The leaves are fanlike with sword-shaped leaf blades. The oval fruits are black and hard with a pale brown covering and a spongy pulp. The taste is soapy and the odor is nutty. Saw palmetto grows in low pinewoods in eastern North America.

Part Used

Fruit

Forms Used

Tincture, standardized extract

Dosage

Tincture: ½ teaspoon (40 drops or 2.5 milliliters) three times a day. Standardized extract: Up to 250 milligrams (95 percent fatty acids) twice a day.

Characteristics

Digestant, antiandrogenic, anti-inflammatory, antihistamine, diuretic, sedative

Cautions

Saw palmetto is generally regarded as safe.

Active Ingredients

Volatile oil, resin, saponins, pectin, mucilage, fatty acids

Use

- Alopecia
- Benign prostatic hyperplasia
- Bladder infection
- Hair thinning or loss
- Impotence

▶ SENNA

Botanical Name

Cassia senna

Other Names

Locust plant, wild senna

Family

Leguminoseae

Description

Senna is native to tropical Africa and is cultivated everywhere. The stem is erect, smooth, and green and bears leaflets in four or five pairs. The leaves are lance-shaped and brittle and have veins on the undersurface. The leaves have a sweet taste and a green tea odor.

Part Used

Leaves

Forms Used

Tea, tablets

Dosage

Tea: 1 tablespoon in one cup water once a day for a maximum of 10 days. Tablets: 50 to 100 milligrams a day.

THE PATIENT FILE

Saw Palmetto Solves Prostate Problems

When John told me that he frequently woke up at night to go to the bathroom, I thought I knew what the problem was. When he told me that he felt as though he never could completely empty his bladder, I was a little more sure. And when he said that a little dribble was the best he could do when he did urinate, I was certain.

John is 55 years old. Like more than half of all men his age, he has an enlarged prostate gland, a condition that's benign but definitely bothersome. The prostate-specific antigen (PSA) test confirmed the diagnosis.

Natural healing has a natural answer for John's condition, and it's not an unnatural pharmaceutical or an invasive surgical procedure. In many instances, supplements can solve the problem.

First off, John needed a good multiple-nutrient supplement that contained at least 30 milligrams of zinc, 1 or 2 milligrams of copper, and 50 milligrams of vitamin B_6. That's just to establish a good nutritional foundation. Next, he needed some extra zinc, so I told him to eat ½ to 1 cup of pumpkin seeds every day. Studies show that eating pumpkin seeds can reduce the incidence of prostate hypertrophy. For added insurance, I told John to swallow a tablespoon of flaxseed oil or evening primrose oil every day and to stop drinking beer. Research links beer drinking to prostate enlargement.

The primary treatment, though, for benign prostate enlargement is a plant—the saw palmetto. I prescribed 160 milligrams twice a day for John. Studies document saw palmetto's ability to shrink enlarged prostate glands just as effectively as and certainly more safely than finasteride, the officially sanctioned prostate-shrinking prescription drug. Men who take saw palmetto urinate more freely, don't awaken as often in the middle of the night to go to the bathroom, and don't experience the erectile inability that plagues their finasteride-taking counterparts.

Soon after John began his nutrient and herb program, he stopped getting up in the middle of the night to urinate. He started to sleep soundly and solidly again. When he goes to the bathroom, he feels as though he's gone to the bathroom. He's fine. His prostate is fine.

Characteristics

Digestant, laxative, stimulant

Cautions

Senna can be habit-forming and therefore should not be used longer than 2 weeks. Long-term use can cause melanosis coli (darkened mucous membranes in the colon). Side effects include diarrhea and gastrointestinal upset. Senna should not be used during pregnancy because it can cause uterine contractions. Senna may inhibit absorption of some drugs, and it can cause albuminuria. It should not be taken by individuals with appendicitis, Crohn's disease, intestinal colic, ulcerative colitis, intestinal inflammation/obstruction, or during lactation, and it should not be used in children under age 10.

Active Ingredients

Anthraquinone, glycosides, flavonoids, volatile oil, resins

Use

- Constipation
- Hemorrhoids

▶ SIBERIAN GINSENG

Botanical Name

Eleutherococcus senticosus

Other Name

Eleuthero

Family

Araliaceae

Description

Ginseng is a perennial herb with a very slow-growing root. The root is a yellowish brown and spindled-shaped and is about 1 inch in diameter, dividing into two or three branches that have a wrinkled appearance. The word *ginseng* means "the wonder of the world."

Part Used

Root

Forms Used

Tincture, capsules, tablets

Dosage

Tincture: ¼ teaspoon (20 drops or 1.3 milliliters) three times a day. Capsules and tablets: 200 to 500 milligrams a day.

Characteristics

Digestant, tonic, immunostimulant, hypoglycemic, circulatory stimulant

Cautions

Siberian ginseng can be too stimulating for some individuals. It can cause insomnia and therefore should not be taken in the evening. Siberian ginseng should not be used by individuals with high blood pressure.

Active Ingredients

Essential oil, saponins, eleuthrosides, polysaccharides

Use

- Adrenal insufficiency
- Aging
- Alzheimer's disease
- Chronic fatigue syndrome
- Coronary heart disease
- Depression
- Fatigue
- Fibromyalgia
- Hepatitis
- HIV infection and AIDS
- Immunodeficiency
- Impotence
- Low blood sugar
- Mononucleosis
- Multiple sclerosis
- Narcolepsy
- Poor concentration/memory
- Radiation exposure

- Stress
- Underactive thyroid

▶ SKULLCAP

Botanical Name

Scutellaria laterifolia

Other Names

Blue pimpernel, blue skullcap, hoodwort, maddog

Family

Labiatae

Description

Skullcap is a perennial with helmet-shaped blue flowers in axillary racemes. The leaves are opposite and lance-shaped. Hybridization with other species often occurs. *Scutellaria laterifolia* species is native to the United States.

Part Used

Whole herb

Forms Used

Tincture, tea

Dosage

Tincture: ½ teaspoon (40 drops or 2.5 milliliters) three times a day. Tea: 1 tablespoon per cup of water; three cups a day.

Characteristics

Sedative, antispasmodic, tonic, astringent, nervine, antibacterial

Cautions

Overdoses of skullcap can cause stimulation of the central nervous system and abnormal heartbeat in some individuals. Skullcap should not be used during pregnancy or lactation. High dosages of skullcap may cause liver damage.

Active Ingredients

Volatile oil, tannins, flavonoids, mucilage, gum

Use

- Anxiety attacks
- Chronic pain
- Fatigue
- Headache
- Insomnia
- Migraine
- Nervousness
- Overactive thyroid
- Palpitations
- Restless legs syndrome

▶ SLIPPERY ELM

Botanical Name

Ulmus rubra

Other Names

Indian elm, moose elm

Family

Ulmaceae

Description

Slippery elm is a small tree (growing to about 60 feet) found in Central and North America and Asia. The bark is deeply furrowed with a ruddy brown color; the inner surface is paler and finely ridged.

Part Used

Bark

Forms Used

Tincture, tea, salve

Dosage

Tincture: ½ teaspoon (40 drops or 2.5 milliliters) three times a day. Tea (decoction): 1 tablespoon per cup of water; two to three cups a day. Salve: Apply topically as needed for burns and wounds.

Characteristics

Demulcent, emollient, astringent

Cautions

Slippery elm is generally regarded as safe.

Active Ingredients

Volatile oil, resin, tannin, mucilage

Use

- Burns
- Colds
- Colic
- Constipation
- Coughs
- Emphysema
- Gastritis
- Heartburn
- Laryngitis
- Peptic ulcer
- Wounds

▶ STAR ANISE

Botanical Name

Illicium verum

Other Name

Chinese anise

Family

Magnoliaceae

Description

Anise is an annual that is native to Egypt and the Mediterranean region and is cultivated in Europe, India, Mexico, Russia, and the United States. The leaves are in long stalks with the lower leaves round and the upper leaves feathery. The leaflets may be toothed or toothless. The fruit is oval and flat with a gray-brown seed.

Part Used

Seeds

Forms Used

Tincture, tea

Dosage

Tincture: ½ teaspoon (40 drops or 2.5 milliliters) three times a day. Tea: 1 tablespoon per cup of water; three cups a day.

Characteristics

Stimulant, carminative, diuretic, digestant, antibacterial, antifungal

Cautions

Star anise is generally regarded as safe. Do not confuse star anise with Japanese star anise, which is poisonous.

Active Ingredients

Volatile oil, trans-anethole

Use

- Colds
- Dyspepsia
- Flatulence
- Fungal infection
- Indigestion
- Morning sickness

▶ STINGING NETTLE

Botanical Name

Urtica dioica

Other Name

Great nettle

Family

Urticaceae

Description

Stinging nettle grows in waste areas everywhere. The whole plant is covered with stinging hairs. The leaves are lance-shaped, opposite, stalked, and finely toothed, tapering to a point. The flowers are green with yellow stamens, and the male and female flowers are on separate plants.

Parts Used

Whole herb, root

Forms Used

Tea, capsules, tablets

Dosage

Tea: 1 tablespoon per cup of water; two to three cups a day. Capsules and tablets: 200 milligrams three times a day.

Characteristics

Anti-inflammatory, digestant, diuretic, hemostatic, antitumor, antiseptic, induces menstruation, expectorant, astringent

Cautions

Stinging nettle can produce allergic reactions in some individuals.

Active Ingredients

Tannin, saponins, lignans, sitosterol, flavonoids, histamine, serotonin, chlorophyll, vitamin C, dietary fiber

Use

- Allergies
- Alopecia
- Asthma
- Benign prostatic hyperplasia
- Burns
- Cancer
- Coughs
- Hair thinning or loss
- Hay fever
- Hives
- Iron-deficiency anemia
- Kidney stones
- Wounds

▶ STRAWBERRY

Botanical Name

Fragaria vesca

Other Names

None

Family

Rosaceae

Description

Strawberry is cultivated worldwide in temperate climates. Strawberry is a thin-leaved plant with small scarlet berries that are cone-shaped and studded with tiny brown seeds. Strawberries are very high in fiber.

Part Used

Leaves

Form Used

Tea

Dosage

1 tablespoon per cup of water; three cups a day. Apply topically for skin disorders.

Characteristics

Astringent, diuretic, uterine tonic

Cautions

Strawberry is generally regarded as safe.

Active Ingredients

Flavonoids, quercetin, tannins, essential oil

Use

- Contact dermatitis
- Diarrhea
- Dysentery
- Eczema

▶ SUMAC

Botanical Name

Rhus glabra

Other Names

Indian salt, smooth sumac

Family

Anacardiaceae

Description

Sumac is a shrub consisting of many straggling branches covered with gray bark. The leaves are green above and white underneath and are alternate and lance-shaped. The flowers are greenish red on spikes, followed by hard red berries. Sumac is abundant in waste areas in the United States and Canada.

Parts Used
Bark, fruit

Form Used
Tincture

Dosage
½ teaspoon (40 drops or 2.5 milliliters) three times a day

Characteristics
Astringent, tonic, antiseptic, diuretic

Cautions
Sumac is generally regarded as safe.

Active Ingredients
Tannins, essential oil, resin

Use
- Diarrhea
- Dysentery
- Fever

▶ SUNFLOWER

Botanical Name
Helianthus annuus

Other Name
Helianthus

Family
Asteraceae

Description
Sunflower is an annual with golden-rayed flowers. The leaves are large, rough, and heart-shaped. The sunflower grows to 15 feet and ranges throughout the world.

Part Used
Seeds

Form Used
Tea (decoction)

Dosage
1 tablespoon per cup of water; two to three cups a day

The Patron Herb of Depression

If you suffer from mild to moderate depression, you could take the drug your doctor prescribes and endure the side effects, or you could effectively elevate your spirits—without side effects—by swallowing supplements of St. John's wort. Americans are only now catching on to what Europeans have long known.

Characteristics
Duretic, expectorant

Cautions
Sunflower is generally regarded as safe.

Active Ingredients
Fixed oil, polyunsaturated fatty acids, protein

Use
- Bronchitis
- Coughs
- Sore throat

▶ SWEET WOODRUFF

Botanical Name
Galium odoratum

Other Names
None

Family
Rubiaceae

Description
Sweet woodruff is a shade-loving perennial ground cover. The leaves are narrow, sword-shaped, and rough-edged, arranged in whorls of six or eight around the stem. The funnel-shaped flowers are white and have four petals. Sweet woodruff is native to Europe and Asia and is cultivated worldwide.

Part Used

Whole herb

Form Used

Tincture

Dosage

½ teaspoon (40 drops or 2.5 milliliters) three times a day

Characteristics

Eases gripping intestinal pain, diuretic, diaphoretic, antispasmodic

Cautions

Sweet woodruff can cause vomiting and dizziness in large doses.

Active Ingredient

Coumarins

Use

- Anxiety attacks
- Indigestion
- Jaundice
- Wounds

▶ TEA TREE

Botanical Name

Melaleuca alternifolia

Other Name

Tea tree oil

Family

Myrtaceae

Description

Tea tree is a small tree native to New South Wales, Australia. The leaves of *Melaleuca alternifolia* were used by early settlers of Australia to make tea, hence the common name. Tea tree oil was used in World War II as a disinfectant.

Part Used

Leaves

Form Used

Essential oil (diluted 50 to 90 percent)

Dosage

Apply to skin three times a day.

Characteristics

Aromatic, antiseptic, antifungal

Cautions

Oral ingestion of tea tree oil is toxic; use only externally. For mouth irritation, apply to affected area and immediately rinse mouth with water. Some individuals may be allergic to tea tree.

Active Ingredients

Volatile oil, terpenes, sesquiterpenes

Use

- Abscesses
- Acne
- Boils
- Burns
- Canker sores
- Cuts and scrapes
- Fungal infection
- Mouth irritation
- Vaginitis

▶ THYME

Botanical Name

Thymus vulgaris

Other Names

Common thyme, garden thyme, mother of thyme, tomillo

Family

Labiatae

Description

Thyme is a perennial shrub. The leaves are opposite, lance-shaped, and hairy, with the edges rolled over. The pink-to-lilac flowers are tubular, occurring in small terminal clusters. Thyme is native to the Mediterranean region and is cultivated worldwide.

Boning Up on Calcium

The best source of calcium is food. Sea vegetables, collard greens, turnip greens, dates, figs, raisins, sesame seeds, kale, celery, rutabagas, soybeans, mustard greens, black strap molasses, dairy products—all are good sources.

Because each of us needs to consume at least 1,200 milligrams of the bone-building mineral per day, though, supplementation can be helpful. But which calcium supplement should you buy? Calcium carbonate, calcium citrate, calcium gluconate? How about calcium lactate or organic chelates of calcium? Does it make a difference?

It does. Some are better absorbed than others.

Calcium is absorbed via your intestines, and stomach acids play a big role in the process. However, many people don't secrete a sufficient amount—at least not enough to sufficiently metabolize the calcium you ingest.

Certain forms of "chelated calcium," particularly calcium citrate but also calcium lactate and calcium gluconate, are best. Calcium carbonate, the most common form sold in stores, is the worst in terms of absorption. If you purchase the cheapest, most readily available calcium supplement, chances are that you're getting calcium carbonate.

If your stomach secretes a "normal" amount of digestive acids, you'll absorb about 22 percent of the calcium in a tablet of calcium carbonate. If your stomach doesn't secrete enough acids, you'll absorb as little as 4 percent. Some 40 percent of postmenopausal women, research shows, are severely deficient in stomach acids. You may be swallowing 1,200 milligrams' worth of calcium every day when, in fact, you're absorbing a mere fraction of that amount.

The good thing about calcium citrate and similar already-ionized forms is that they're available for absorption as soon as you swallow the tablets. People with low levels of stomach acid who ingest calcium citrate supplements absorb about 45 percent of this valuable mineral immediately.

▶ In the face of many conflicting reports, chances are that each form of a nutrient is just as good as other forms.

▶ If only the manufacturer is touting a certain form as superior to all others, you can usually discount the claim. One exception is high-selenium yeast. Right now, only one company provides this nutrient to all other distributors.

▶ Do not forget to read labels carefully. You need to know precisely what form of any nutrient you are consuming. You can contact the manufacturer for documentation about the benefits of taking their products.

HOW TO USE THE VITAMINS, MINERALS, AND SUPPLEMENTS SECTION OF THIS BOOK

This section covers more than 80 popular vitamins, minerals, and supplements (referred to, collectively, as "supplements"). Each entry includes a description, the form or forms used, dosages, and precautions. You'll also find a list of foods containing these substances, along with useful combinations of supplements and other natural medicines or pharmaceuticals that can enhance health benefits.

IMPORTANT PRECAUTIONS

You should not take supplements to treat a health condition without consulting a physician beforehand. Accurate diagnosis is vital in order to undertake an appropriate course of treatment. If you are pregnant or contemplating pregnancy, or if you are currently taking medication to treat an illness or condition, you should be particularly careful to seek medical advice before undertaking a supplement regimen (see Supplements and Safety Precautions, on pages 250-252).

Dosages given in this book represent the safe daily intake for average adults. Children and the elderly may require different dosages, and dosage amounts may vary depending on a variety of factors, including age, body weight, and type of health condition (see Dosages, on pages 252-254).

A KEY TO USES

Each vitamin, mineral, or supplement described in this section of the book is accompanied by a list of potential uses. This list specifies the health conditions for which a supplement may be particularly beneficial or appropriate. Each chart includes a T, P, or B designation.

T—Can be used *therapeutically* to help treat a disease or condition once it has occurred. Vitamin E, for example, can be helpful in treating acne.

P—Can be used to help *prevent* a disease or condition from occurring. Folic acid, for example, is helpful in preventing birth defects.

B—Can be used to help *both* in prevention and treatment. Iron, for example, is useful in both preventing and treating anemia brought on by iron deficiency.

The T, P, and B designations are based on the author's clinical experience, on how the supplement affects body function, and on scientific research, when available. It is important to qualify them, however.

In some cases, research supports a direct health benefit that can be derived from using a particular supplement. In other cases, no direct health benefit can be demonstrated, but the supplement may play a peripheral role in preventing or treating a particular health condition. For example, not much research is available on the role of calcium in the treatment of angina, anxiety, or arrhythmia, although we do know that calcium helps regulate the heartbeat. Much of this information is based on the author's clinical experience treating many of these health conditions.

▶ ACETYL-L-CARNITINE

Abbreviation

ALC

Other Name

L-carnitine

Description

Needed to move fatty acids into cell mitochondria and used for energy, carnitine is made from the amino acids lysine and methionine. Symptoms of deficiency include progressive muscle weakness and buildup of fats in skeletal muscles, heart muscle, and liver. This carnitine form may help delay progression of Alzheimer's.

Forms Used

Capsules, tablets

Dosage

500 to 2,000 milligrams a day

Useful Combinations

Iron, niacin (vitamin B_3), vitamin B_6, and vitamin C are required by the body to convert the amino acids lysine and methionine to carnitine. Carnitine appears to work synergistically with coenzyme Q_{10}.

Cautions

None known

Signs of Overdose

Anxiety, agitation, restlessness, skin rash, nausea, vomiting

Food Sources

Chicken, beef, seafood, turkey, nuts, seeds, dairy products

Use

Disorder	T	P	B
Alzheimer's disease	✓		
Depression	✓		
Down syndrome	✓		

▶ ALANINE

Abbreviation

Ala

Other Name

L-alanine

Description

Alanine is a nonessential amino acid that aids the metabolism of glucose. Alanine is also a constituent of vitamin B_5 (pantothenic acid) and coenzyme A, a vital catalyst in the body. Alanine is needed for proper function of the prostate gland.

Forms Used

Capsules, tablets, powder

Dosage

500 to 1,000 milligrams a day

Useful Combinations

None known

Cautions

Individuals with kidney or liver damage should consult a physician before taking alanine, as supplementing with amino acids can cause further damage to these organs.

Signs of Overdose

None known

Food Sources

Seafood, turkey, chicken, pork, beef, eggs, beans, nuts, seeds

Use

Disorder	T	P	B
Adrenal insufficiency	✓		
Benign prostatic hyperplasia	✓		
Depression	✓		
Diabetes	✓		
Seizures	✓		

T=Therapeutic **P**=Preventive **B**=Both

▶ ARGININE

Abbreviation

Arg

Other Name

L-arginine

Description

Arginine is a nonessential amino acid involved in the synthesis of urea, a waste product from protein metabolism, and creatine. Studies have shown that arginine supplementation may be beneficial in cases of infection and wound healing because it stimulates the immune system. Arginine supplementation may also increase sperm counts in infertile men. Arginine may decrease platelet aggregation and reduce blood pressure and cholesterol levels.

Forms Used

Capsules, tablets, powder

Dosage

1 to 2 grams a day

Useful Combinations

Lysine offsets the pro-herpes effect of arginine; it has been shown to inhibit replication of the herpesvirus. Therefore, a diet high in lysine and low in arginine is recommended.

Cautions

Avoid arginine supplementation if you have herpes simplex, peptic ulcer, pseudomonas bacterial infections, or severe liver or kidney disease.

Signs of Overdose

Herpes outbreak, diarrhea

Food Sources

Seafood, turkey, chicken, dairy products, pork, beef, eggs, beans, nuts, seeds, peanuts, chocolate, whole grains, carob, raisins

Use

Disorder	T	P	B
Angina	✓		
Cancer	✓		
Colds		✓	
Congestive heart failure	✓		
High blood pressure	✓		
High cholesterol levels	✓		
Immunodeficiency	✓		
Male infertility	✓		
Wounds	✓		

▶ ASPARTIC ACID

Abbreviation

Asp

Other Names

Aspartate, L-aspartic acid, potassium-magnesium aspartate

Description

Aspartic acid is an amino acid and neurotransmitter in the brain. Aspartate feeds into the Krebs cycle, which is the final pathway for the conversion of glucose, fatty acids, and amino acids into energy, or ATP (adenosine 5-triphosphate). Studies show that minerals are absorbed better if they are bound to aspartate or other Krebs cycle intermediates (malate, citrate, or succinate). Aspartic acid has been shown to increase stamina and help detoxify the liver.

Forms Used

Capsules, tablets, powder

Dosage

1 to 2 grams a day

Useful Combinations

Vitamin B_6 is essential for metabolizing aspartate.

Cautions

Use with caution in epilepsy and stroke because aspartic acid is a neurotransmitter in the brain.

T=Therapeutic   **P**=Preventive   **B**=Both

Signs of Overdose

Nausea, diarrhea, sedation (rare), loss of motivation (rare), infertility (rare)

Food Sources

Seafood, turkey, chicken, pork, beef, eggs, beans, nuts, seeds

Use

Disorder	T	P	B
Abnormal heartbeat	✓		
Congestive heart failure	✓		
Coronary heart disease	✓		
Depression	✓		
Fatigue	✓		
Male infertility	✓		
Palpitations	✓		
Radiation exposure	✓		

▶ BETA-CAROTENE

Abbreviation

Pro-Vit-A

Other Name

Provitamin A

Description

Beta-carotene is a precursor to vitamin A. Beta-carotene is an antioxidant, meaning it protects cells against oxygen damage, and it is commonly used to help prevent cancer and cardiovascular disease. Beta-carotene has also been shown to stimulate the immune system. Food sources of carotenoids can usually be identified by their yellow or red-orange color; for example, carrots, yellow squash, and apricots are high in beta-carotene.

Forms Used

Capsules, tablets, liquid

Dosage

25,000 international units a day

Useful Combinations

Beta-carotene is best taken with other carotenoids (alpha-carotene, lutein, lycopene)

and vitamin E. Beta-carotene taken with iron may enhance iron absorption. Deficiencies of protein, thyroid hormone, vitamin C, or zinc may impair the conversion of beta-carotene to vitamin A.

Cautions

Some people develop orange palms when taking high doses of beta-carotene. Pregnant women should not take more than 5,000 international units a day of beta-carotene because it can cause birth defects.

Signs of Overdose

Loss of menstrual period (amenorrhea), underactive thyroid, hair loss, bone pain, headache

Food Sources

Spinach, mustard greens, liver, chili peppers, dandelion root, collard greens, sweet potatoes, carrots, green beans, other dark green or orange vegetables, orange fruits

Use

Disorder	T	P	B
Aging		✓	
Autoimmune disease			✓
Breast cancer			✓
Cataracts	✓		
Cervical dysplasia	✓		
Colorectal cancer			✓
Congestive heart failure		✓	
Contact dermatitis	✓		
Coronary heart disease			✓
Crohn's disease	✓		
Down syndrome	✓		
Dry eyes	✓		
High cholesterol			✓
HIV infection and AIDS	✓		
Immunodeficiency	✓		
Lung cancer			✓
Lupus	✓		
Macular degeneration		✓	
Menopausal symptoms	✓		
Night blindness	✓		
Skin cancer			✓
Stomach cancer			✓
Surgery recovery	✓		
Vaginitis	✓		

T=Therapeutic **P**=Preventive **B**=Both

THE PATIENT FILE

From a Cold to a Cancer to a Cure

Christine had a cold the first time I met her. In fact, that's why she came to see me. I soon learned, though, that a cold was the least of her concerns.

During our conversation, I discovered that the 32-year-old woman had, a year earlier, an abnormal Pap smear, which can indicate cervical cancer. I ordered the pathology report and learned that she indeed had cervical dysplasia, a condition that often heralds the development of cancer.

Christine never returned to the physician who performed the Pap smear because she didn't like the way she was treated. She felt threatened, she told me, and no one in the doctor's office had bothered to explain in simple terms the threat that confronted her. Apparently feeling challenged and ill at ease, she chose simply to retreat and concede defeat.

I began treatment by cautioning Christine about several major lifestyle contributions to cervical cancer, specifically smoking, using oral contraceptives, and entertaining several sex partners. Then I honed in on the dietary culprits. She needed to eat at least five different vegetables and three different fruits every day of her life. She also needed to stop eating red meat.

Last, she needed a big boost in her supplemental intake. I prescribed a daily dosage of 100,000 international units of beta-carotene, 10 milligrams of folic acid, 100 micrograms of selenium, 50,000 international units of vitamin A, 100 milligrams of vitamin B$_6$, and 400 international units of vitamin E.

In 2 months, Christine returned to my office for another Pap smear. No signs of dysplasia! I told her to come back in 3 months. She did. We retested and you can guess the outcome. Her cold had gone away long before, too.

▶ BIOTIN

Abbreviation

None

Other Name

Biocytin

Description

Biotin is a water-soluble B vitamin. It is important in the synthesis of glucose, fatty acids, and DNA and in the metabolism of certain amino acids. Biotin deficiency may cause nausea, thinning hair, loss of hair color, skin rash, depression, lethargy, hallucinations, and tingling of the extremities.

Forms Used

Capsules, powder, liquid

Dosage

3 to 30 micrograms a day

Useful Combinations

Biotin is best absorbed when combined with B-complex vitamins, folic acid, and zinc. Carnitine and coenzyme Q$_{10}$ work synergistically with biotin.

Cautions

Alcohol and antibiotics may inhibit the absorption of biotin.

Signs of Overdose

An excess of one B vitamin may cause a deficiency in the other B vitamins. Therefore,

---

T=Therapeutic **P**=Preventive **B**=Both

biotin should be taken in combination with a B-complex vitamin.

Food Sources

Brewer's yeast, liver, soybeans, rice, egg yolks, peanuts, walnuts, barley, pecans, oatmeal, sardines, black-eyed peas, split peas, almonds, cauliflower, mushrooms

Use

Disorder	T	P	B
Cradle cap	✓		
Dandruff	✓		
Depression	✓		
Diabetes	✓		
Diabetic neuropathy	✓		
Dialysis		✓	
Dry skin	✓		
Growth retardation		✓	
Hair thinning or loss	✓		
Osteoporosis			✓
Renal failure	✓		
Weak fingernails	✓		

▶ BORON

Abbreviation

B

Other Names

Boron aspartate, boron chelate, boron citrate, boron gluconate

Description

Boron is a mineral involved in calcium, potassium, magnesium, and vitamin D metabolism. Boron is important for the maintenance of healthy bones and proper joint function.

Forms Used

Capsules, tablets

Dosage

1 to 9 milligrams a day

Useful Combinations

Boron may act synergistically with calcium, magnesium, vitamin D, and other nutrients for the treatment of osteoporosis.

Cautions

None known

Signs of Overdose

Nausea, vomiting, abdominal pain, rash, convulsions

Food Sources

Fruits, vegetables, nuts

Use

Disorder	T	P	B
Fractured bone			✓
Osteoarthritis		✓	
Osteoporosis		✓	
Rheumatoid arthritis		✓	

▶ BROMELAIN

Abbreviation

None

Other Name

Enzymes derived from pineapple stems

Description

Bromelain is a proteolytic enzyme made from the pineapple plant. Bromelain has been shown to have anti-inflammatory effects and to enhance wound repair. Also, it is a digestive aid and a smooth-muscle relaxer.

Forms Used

Capsules, tablets

Dosage

Inflammation and wounds: 500 milligrams three times a day between meals. Digestion: 500 milligrams three times a day, with meals.

Useful Combinations

Curcumin enhances bromelain's anti-inflammatory effects. Bromelain enhances the effects of digestive enzymes such as papain, lipase, and proteases. Bromelain may increase the absorption of some antibiotics, such as amoxicillin.

T=Therapeutic   **P**=Preventive   **B**=Both

Cautions

Individuals with high blood pressure should consult a physician before taking bromelain. Some individuals may be allergic to bromelain. Because bromelain acts as a blood thinner, it may react with blood-thinning medications, possibly causing excessive bleeding.

Signs of Overdose

Hypertensive individuals may experience tachycardia from taking high doses of bromelain.

Food Source

Pineapple

Use

Disorder	T	P	B
Abscesses	✓		
Allergies	✓		
Angina	✓		
Appetite loss	✓		
Asthma	✓		
Bad breath	✓		
Carpal tunnel syndrome	✓		
Celiac disease	✓		
Chronic pain	✓		
Contact dermatitis	✓		
Crohn's disease	✓		
Flatulence	✓		
Fluid retention or swelling	✓		
Hay fever	✓		
Heartburn	✓		
Hives	✓		
Indigestion	✓		
Inflammation	✓		
Joint pain	✓		
Lower-back pain	✓		
Lymph node swelling	✓		
Morning sickness	✓		
Muscle strain	✓		
Nausea	✓		
Neuralgia and neuritis	✓		
Osteoarthritis	✓		
Rheumatoid arthritis	✓		
Sinusitis	✓		
Sprains	✓		
Surgery recovery		✓	
Varicose veins		✓	
Wounds	✓		

▶ CALCIUM

Abbreviation

Ca

Other Names

Calcium carbonate, calcium chelate, calcium citrate, calcium gluconate, calcium lactate, calcium malate, calcium microcrystalline hydroxyapatite, calcium phosphate

Description

Calcium is the most abundant mineral in the body. Ninety-nine percent of the body's calcium is found in bones and teeth. The other 1 percent is in soft tissues and body fluids and is essential for proper nerve and muscle function, regulation of the heartbeat, and blood clotting. Calcium may regulate blood pressure by controlling the contraction of muscles in the blood vessel walls and by signaling the secretion of blood pressure regulators. Inadequate calcium absorption can result in rickets (stunted bone growth) in children and osteoporosis (porous, fragile bones) or osteomalacia (soft bones) in adults.

Forms Used

Capsules, tablets, powder, liquid

Dosage

500 to 1,500 milligrams per day

Useful Combinations

Calcium is best taken in combination with magnesium, vitamin K, boron, and vitamin D.

Cautions

Calcium interferes with the absorption of antibiotics such as tetracycline and ciprofloxacin as well as iron and zinc. Antibiotics may decrease calcium absorption. Calcium may potentiate digitalis toxicity. Histamine-2 blockers,

T=Therapeutic   P=Preventive   B=Both

such as Tagamet, Zantac, Pepcid, and Axid, and related drugs, such as Prilosec, reduce gastric acidity and may reduce absorption of calcium, folic acid, iron, magnesium, vitamin B_{12}, and zinc. Too much calcium may cause constipation. Individuals with hyperparathyroidism and hypercalcemia should not take calcium. Corticosteroid use has been associated with osteoporosis and a depletion of calcium. Caffeine, alcohol, phosphates, protein, sodium, sugar, and aluminum-containing antacids all may decrease calcium absorption.

Signs of Overdose

Constipation, muscle spasms, gas, bloating, calcium kidney stones

Food Sources

Kelp, Swiss cheese, Cheddar cheese, carob flour, collard greens, turnip greens

Use

Disorder	T	P	B
Abnormal heartbeat	✓		
Aluminum poisoning	✓		
Angina	✓		
Anxiety attacks	✓		
Bipolar disorder		✓	
Breastfeeding complications		✓	
Cardiomyopathy	✓		
Carpal tunnel syndrome	✓		
Cavities and tooth decay			✓
Chondromalacia	✓		
Chronic fatigue syndrome	✓		
Chronic pain	✓		
Colorectal cancer		✓	
Congestive heart failure	✓		
Coronary heart disease			✓
Corticosteroid therapy	✓		
Crohn's disease	✓		
Depression	✓		
Disk problems	✓		
Emphysema	✓		
Fatigue	✓		
Fractured bone			✓
Growth retardation	✓		
Gum disease	✓		
Headache	✓		
Heart attack		✓	

Natural Regimen for Menstrual Cramps

Mary, 28, had cramps during her menstrual periods for about 5 years. Aspirin and ibuprofen had helped, until the past year. The cramps had become very painful, and they were worse on her right side.

Mary's menstrual flow for the first few days was heavy and clotted. She felt as though something were bearing down on her pelvic organs, especially when she moved around; she felt better when lying in bed. Some days, she was extremely thirsty for cold water; other days, she wasn't thirsty at all. The lab test showed no cysts, fibroids, or endometriosis. Because of her symptoms, I recommended that she take a 30C Belladonna pill every 15 minutes for an hour until her pain resolved. I also prescribed yoga stretching exercises.

I advised her to take a daily supplement regimen of 1,200 milligrams calcium citrate, 600 milligrams magnesium citrate, and 1 tablespoon organic flaxseed oil. Further, Mary was to avoid alcohol, caffeine, and salt and eat five kinds of vegetables and three kinds of fruits daily. One month later, Mary returned to report that her menstrual cramps were gone.

To keep the problem from recurring, I suggested that she continue the supplement regimen, the yoga stretches, and the revised diet.

Disorder	T	P	B
Heart murmurs	✓		
Hemorrhoids	✓		
High blood pressure	✓		
High cholesterol levels	✓		
Insomnia	✓		

T=Therapeutic   **P**=Preventive   **B**=Both

Disorder	T	P	B
Intermittent claudication	✓		
Kidney stones		✓	
Leg cramps	✓		
Lower-back pain	✓		
Lupus	✓		
Magnesium therapy	✓		
Menopausal symptoms		✓	
Menstrual cramps	✓		
Menstrual period cessation	✓		
Migraine	✓		
Mitral valve prolapse	✓		
Multiple sclerosis	✓		
Muscle strain	✓		
Myasthenia gravis	✓		
Osteoporosis		✓	
Overactive thyroid		✓	
Palpitations	✓		
Periodontal disease	✓		
Pregnancy complications	✓		
Premenstrual syndrome	✓		
Restless legs syndrome	✓		
Schizophrenia		✓	
Sprains	✓		
Tinnitus	✓		
Ulcerative colitis		✓	

▶ CARNITINE

Abbreviation

None

Other Name

L-carnitine

Description

Made from the amino acids lysine and methionine, carnitine is needed to move fatty acids into cell mitochondria and is used for energy. Symptoms of deficiency include progressive muscle weakness with buildup of fats in skeletal muscles, heart muscle, and liver. This carnitine form is used mainly for heart conditions.

Forms Used

Capsules, tablets

Dosage

500 to 4,000 milligrams a day

Useful Combinations

Carnitine may lower the toxicity of valproic acid, pivampicillin, emetine, sulfadiazine, and pyrimethamine. Carnitine may also protect the heart from the damage that sometimes occurs in people using the chemotherapy drug Adriamycin (doxorubicin hydrochloride). Carnitine works synergistically with coenzyme Q_{10} and vitamin B_5 (pantothenic acid).

Cautions

Carnitine may cause heartburn. There are no known combinations to avoid or other contraindications.

Signs of Overdose

Heartburn, elevated cholesterol (rare)

Food Sources

Chicken, beef, seafood, turkey, nuts, seeds

Use

Disorder	T	P	B
Abnormal heartbeat	✓		
Angina	✓		
Capillary fragility	✓		
Cardiomyopathy	✓		
Cirrhosis	✓		
Congestive heart failure	✓		
Coronary heart disease	✓		
Diabetes	✓		
Diabetic neuropathy	✓		
Emphysema	✓		
Exercise endurance		✓	
Fibromyalgia	✓		
Heart attack	✓		
Heart murmurs	✓		
High cholesterol levels	✓		
Impaired exercise performance	✓		
Intermittent claudication	✓		
Low blood sugar	✓		
Male infertility	✓		
Mitral valve prolapse	✓		
Palpitations	✓		
Poor concentration/memory	✓		
Renal failure	✓		

T=Therapeutic   **P**=Preventive   **B**=Both

▶ CETYL MYRISTOLEATE

Abbreviation

None

Other Name

cis-9-cetyl myristoleate

Description

Cetyl myristoleate is an oil and ester of the unsaturated fatty acid cis-9-tetradecanoic acid. As a fatty acid ester, cetyl myristoleate has been shown to have anti-inflammatory properties.

Forms Used

Capsules, tablets

Dosage

1 to 5 grams a day

Useful Combinations

Useful combinations include glucosamine sulfate, fish oil, flaxseed oil, vitamin E, and curcumin.

Cautions

To maximize absorption, avoid colas, citrus juices, sugar, alcohol, and caffeine. Cetyl myristoleate should not be used by pregnant or lactating women.

Signs of Overdose

None known

Food Source

Myristoleic acid is found in fish oils, whale oils, and kombu butter.

Use

Disorder	T	P	B
Osteoarthritis	✓		
Rheumatoid arthritis	✓		

▶ CHOLINE

Abbreviation

None

Other Names

Lecithin, phosphatidylcholine

Description

Choline is needed to manufacture the neurotransmitter acetylcholine. Acetylcholine is needed for proper nervous-system function and is also a main component of cell membranes in the form of phosphatidylcholine, or lecithin. Choline is an essential nutrient because it is needed for proper metabolism of fats. It can be manufactured in the human body from either the amino acid methionine or the amino acid serine.

Forms Used

Capsules, tablets

Dosage

500 to 1,000 milligrams a day

Useful Combinations

None known

Cautions

High doses of choline can cause disagreeable body odor and can potentiate the toxicity of morphine. In general use, choline can cause a fishy odor, whereas phosphatidylcholine does not. Do not use choline with anticholinergic drugs.

Signs of Overdose

Depression can be a sign of overdose. Side effects may include diarrhea, excessive sweating, nausea, and gastrointestinal problems.

Food Sources

Lecithin, egg yolks, liver, wheat germ, soybeans, rice, black-eyed peas, garbanzo beans, brewer's yeast, lentils, split peas, peanuts, oatmeal, barley, ham, whole wheat, molasses, pork, beef, green peas, sweet potatoes

T=Therapeutic   **P**=Preventive   **B**=Both

The Natural Blend

The components of natural healing often blend beautifully with one another to restore health without the need for prescription medications. Just ask Jan, a 48-year-old woman who had been sweating through heart palpitations and anxiety attacks for 3 years.

The divorce Jan was going through could have been a main source of her physical problems, but I suspected something more was in play. When she told me that her menstrual periods had been sporadic for the last year or so and that she was experiencing hot flashes, the answer seemed pretty obvious: Jan was perimenopausal. The heart palpitations, the anxiety, the hot flashes—all were prompted by her body's hormone shifts.

I did not prescribe hormone replacement therapy because it can significantly raise a woman's risk for breast and uterine cancer. Though prescription hormones can reduce the chance of osteoporosis, Jan already was at low risk for this disease. She exercised, took supplements of calcium citrate (1,200 milligrams) and magnesium citrate (600 milligrams) every day, and did not eat meat.

Instead of drugs, Jan needed to beef up her diet and revise her supplement strategy. For more bone-building protection as well as to reduce her risk of breast cancer and help regulate the hot flashes, I told her to eat more soy, including 150 milligrams of soy isoflavones daily. I also recommended that she take a tablespoon of flaxseed oil daily.

I also suggested that she regularly ingest a tincture composed of 3 parts black cohosh, 2 parts dong quai, 2 parts hawthorn, and 1 part passionflower. Hawthorn and passionflower help ease anxiety and quell palpitations.

A month later, Jan felt much better. The hot flashes had cooled considerably and the palpitations had eased up. She still had them occasionally, but they weren't quite so dreadful. The only change I made to her therapy was the addition of 30 milligrams of the heart-helping nutrient coenzyme Q_{10} (CoQ_{10}) twice a day. It was the finishing touch on a comprehensive natural approach to ending Jan's nagging health problems.

Thirty days later, I called Jan to check up on her. She hadn't had a single palpitation since starting the CoQ_{10}.

Use

Disorder	T	P	B
Alcoholism	✓		
Alzheimer's disease	✓		
Cirrhosis	✓		
Growth retardation		✓	
Headache	✓		
Heavy metal toxicity	✓		
Hepatitis	✓		
Myasthenia gravis	✓		
Seizures	✓		
Tardive dyskinesia	✓		

T=Therapeutic   **P**=Preventive   **B**=Both

▶ CHROMIUM

Abbreviation

Cr

Other Names

Chromium aspartate, chromium citrate, chromium picolinate, chromium polynicotinate

Description

Chromium is an important mineral in the regulation of blood sugar and insulin levels. Chromium supplementation can also reduce sugar cravings. Intake of simple sugars, intake of refined carbohydrates such as white flour, and strenuous exercise can deplete chromium.

Forms Used

Capsules, tablets

Dosage

200 to 400 micrograms a day

Useful Combinations

Chromium and low-dose niacin are synergistic in lowering blood cholesterol levels. Vitamin C may increase the absorption of chromium.

Cautions

High doses of chromium should not be used by individuals with kidney or liver disease.

Signs of Overdose

None known

Food Sources

Brewer's yeast, beef, liver, whole wheat, rye, oysters, potatoes, green peppers, eggs, chicken, apples, butter, parsnips, corn, lamb, scallops, Swiss cheese, bananas, spinach

Use

Disorder	T	P	B
Acne		✓	
Adrenal insufficiency	✓		
Alcoholism	✓		
Anorexia nervosa	✓		
Anxiety attacks	✓		
Coronary heart disease			✓
Diabetes	✓		
Glaucoma	✓		
High blood sugar	✓		
High cholesterol levels	✓		
Low blood sugar	✓		
Morning sickness	✓		
Obesity	✓		

▶ COENZYME Q₁₀

Abbreviations

Q_{10}, CoQ_{10}

Other Name

Ubiquinone

Description

Coenzyme Q_{10} is an important component of cell mitochondria, which are small, energy-producing structures located in the cell cytoplasm. Coenzyme Q_{10} is also involved in the manufacture of adenosine 5-triphosphate (ATP), the energy source of all body functions. Coenzyme Q_{10} is an essential nutrient for normal heart function and immune system support, and it can be helpful as a supplement for individuals with gum disease or overactive thyroid glands.

Form Used

Capsules

Dosage

50 to 360 milligrams a day

Useful Combinations

CoQ_{10} lowers the toxicity of Adriamycin (a chemotherapy drug) and lovastatin (a cholesterol-lowering drug) and can counteract some of the side effects of beta-blockers (propranolol, nadolol, atenolol, timolol) and psychotropic drugs (phenothiazines and tricyclic antidepressants).

Cautions

Lovastatin, pravastatin, simvastatin, and other drugs that inhibit HMG-COA (3 hydroxy 3-methylglutaryl-coenzyme A) may deplete coenzyme Q_{10} levels in the body.

Signs of Overdose

None known

T=Therapeutic   **P**=Preventive   **B**=Both

Dosage

Up to 1,000 milligrams twice a day, taken 20 minutes before meals

Useful Combinations

Use of quercetin is beneficial during chemotherapy and radiation therapy. Quercetin enhances the effects of bromelain, curcumin, and vitamin C.

Cautions

Do not use high doses of quercetin on a long-term basis.

Sign of Overdose

Stomach upset

Food Sources

Citrus fruits, berries, onions, legumes, green tea, red wine

Use

Disorder	T	P	B
Allergies			✓
Asthma	✓		
Cancer			✓
Capillary fragility	✓		
Carpal tunnel syndrome	✓		
Cataracts	✓		
Chronic pain	✓		
Conjunctivitis	✓		
Contact dermatitis	✓		
Coronary heart disease		✓	
Crohn's disease	✓		
Diabetic neuropathy	✓		
Down syndrome	✓		
Eczema	✓		
Fibrocystic breasts	✓		
Fluid retention or swelling	✓		
Hay fever	✓		
Hives	✓		
HIV infection and AIDS	✓		
Inflammation	✓		
Joint pain	✓		
Lower-back pain	✓		
Migraine	✓		
Muscle strain	✓		
Neuralgia and neuritis	✓		
Osteoarthritis	✓		
Psoriasis	✓		
Rheumatoid arthritis	✓		

Disorder	T	P	B
Sinusitis	✓		
Sprains	✓		
Surgery recovery		✓	
Ulcerative colitis	✓		

▶ S-ADENOSYL-METHIONINE

Abbreviation

SAM

Other Names

Methionine, SAM-E

Description

S-adenosylmethionine is a nutrient that is produced in the body by the combination of the essential amino acid methionine with ATP (adenosine 5-triphosphate). As a methyl donor, SAM is involved in the production of DNA, RNA, proteins, certain vitamins, neurotransmitters, antioxidants, hormones, and phospholipids and is part of the detoxification process. Because of SAM's vital role in many biochemical pathways, it has been shown to support brain chemistry and joint and connective tissue function and to be effective against various liver disorders. Tissue levels of SAM are typically low in the elderly and in patients with osteoarthritis, depression, or liver disease.

Forms Used

Capsules, tablets

Dosage

800 to 1,600 milligrams a day

Useful Combinations

SAM may increase the effects of antidepressants.

Cautions

S-adenosylmethionine should not be used by individuals with high levels of homocysteine in

T=Therapeutic   **P**=Preventive   **B**=Both

the blood or by those consuming alcohol. Individuals with bipolar depression should not take SAM because its antidepressant activity may lead to a manic state. SAM may be used with other types of depression, however.

Signs of Overdose

Gastrointestinal upset, nausea

Food Sources

Chicken, beef, seafood, turkey, nuts, seeds

Use

Disorder	T	P	B
Bile flow obstruction	✓		
Cirrhosis	✓		
Depression	✓		
Fibromyalgia	✓		
Hepatitis	✓		
Obesity	✓		
Osteoarthritis	✓		
Parkinson's disease	✓		
Rheumatoid arthritis	✓		

▶ SELENIUM

Abbreviation

Se

Other Names

Selenium citrate, selenium picolinate, selenocysteine, selenomethionine, sodium selenite

Description

Selenium interacts with vitamin E and other antioxidants to protect the body against oxidative stress. It is an essential part of the enzyme glutathione peroxidase, which breaks down free radicals. Selenium is also needed for the synthesis of thyroid hormones. Selenium deficiency has been seen in individuals living in certain parts of China where the soil is deficient in selenium and all the food is grown locally. Symptoms of selenium deficiency include muscular discomfort, weakness, and a form of heart disease called Keshan disease.

Forms Used

Capsules, tablets

Dosage

100 to 200 micrograms a day

Useful Combinations

Selenium works with vitamin E to prevent free-radical damage to cell membranes.

Cautions

High doses of selenium taken for long periods are toxic. Large doses may cause skin rashes or neurological problems. Avoid high intake of alcohol with selenium.

Signs of Overdose

Skin rash, neurological problems, metal taste, fatigue, hair loss, weakness, loss of appetite, headache

Food Sources

Butter, herring, smelt, wheat germ, Brazil nuts, pumpkin seeds, apple cider vinegar, scallops, barley, whole wheat, lobster, bran, shrimp, Swiss chard, oats, clams, king crab, oysters, milk, cod, brown rice, beef, lamb, turnips, molasses, garlic, barley

Use

Disorder	T	P	B
Aging		✓	
Autoimmune disease		✓	
Breast cancer			✓
Cancer		✓	
Cataracts			✓
Cervical dysplasia	✓		
Chondromalacia	✓		
Cirrhosis	✓		
Colorectal cancer		✓	
Congestive heart failure	✓		
Coronary heart disease		✓	
Crohn's disease			✓
Dandruff	✓		
Down syndrome	✓		
Emphysema	✓		
Growth retardation	✓		
Heart attack		✓	
High blood pressure		✓	
High cholesterol levels	✓		

T=Therapeutic   **P**=Preventive   **B**=Both

Disorder	T	P	B
HIV infection and AIDS	✓		
Immunodeficiency	✓		
Intermittent claudication	✓		
Leg ulcers	✓		
Lung cancer	✓		
Lupus		✓	
Macular degeneration			✓
Male infertility		✓	
Menopausal symptoms			✓
Multiple sclerosis	✓		
Mumps		✓	
Muscular dystrophy	✓		
Osgood-Schlatter disease	✓		
Overactive thyroid		✓	
Seizures	✓		
Skin cancer	✓		
Stomach cancer	✓		

▶ SHARK CARTILAGE

Abbreviation

None

Other Name

Cartilage

Description

Shark cartilage is a form of connective tissue that is composed of mucopolysaccharides, protein, calcium, and collagen. Studies have shown that shark cartilage may have a role in inhibiting tumor growth by stimulating the immune system and inhibiting angiogenesis (growth of new blood vessels) in tumors. There are also bovine sources of cartilage.

Forms Used

Capsules, tablets

Dosage

1 to 5 grams a day, taken 30 minutes before meals

Useful Combinations

Shark cartilage is better absorbed when taken with calcium or bicarbonate.

Cautions

Do not take shark cartilage if you are pregnant or nursing.

Signs of Overdose

None known

Food Source

Shark

Use

Disorder	T	P	B
Cancer	✓		
Osteoarthritis	✓		
Rheumatoid arthritis	✓		

▶ SILICON

Abbreviation

Si

Other Name

None

Description

Silicon is involved in the synthesis of collagen and the calcification of bone. Silicon aids in collagen cross-linking and in the initiation of bone mineralization. Animal studies have shown that silicon deficiency in animals has resulted in abnormalities in bone and connective tissue.

Forms Used

Capsules, tablets, liquid

Dosage

10 to 40 micrograms a day

Useful Combinations

None known

Cautions

Large doses of silicon taken long-term may be associated with Alzheimer's disease.

Signs of Overdose

None known

T=Therapeutic   P=Preventive   B=Both

Food Sources

Oatmeal, brown rice, root vegetables

Use

Disorder	T	P	B
Coronary heart disease		✓	
Osteoporosis		✓	

▶ SODIUM

Abbreviation

Na

Other Names

Bicarbonate, iodized salt, sea salt, sodium citrate, sodium glutamate

Description

As an electrolyte, sodium helps regulate fluid balance and nerve conduction in the body. Sodium is the most abundant electrolyte outside the cells and is therefore the primary regulator of extracellular fluid volume. The kidneys are the primary regulator of sodium concentration in the body. Urinary excretion of sodium is decreased when sodium intake is low and increased when sodium intake is high. Because water follows sodium by osmosis, the ability of the kidneys to conserve salt provides a mechanism to conserve body water. When sodium concentration increases, water follows, causing an increase in the volume of extracellular fluid in the blood. Changes in blood volume can increase or decrease blood pressure. Changes in blood pressure trigger the production and release of proteins and hormones that affect the amount of sodium and water retained by the kidneys.

Forms Used

Tablets, powder

Dosage

Less than 1,000 milligrams a day

Useful Combinations

None known

Cautions

Use sodium in strict moderation if you have high blood pressure, kidney stones, osteoporosis, stroke, or congestive heart failure.

Signs of Overdose

High blood pressure, fluid retention or swelling

Food Sources

Kelp, green olives, dill pickles, sauerkraut, Cheddar cheese, scallops, cottage cheese, salt

Use

Disorder	T	P	B
Heat exhaustion	✓		
Heatstroke	✓		
Leg cramps	✓		
Low blood pressure	✓		

▶ TAURINE

Abbreviation

None

Other Name

None

Description

Taurine is an amino acid that is necessary for nerve function and vision and is a component of bile salts. Taurine is synthesized from either methionine or cysteine, both of which are amino acids. Taurine regulates the heartbeat, platelet aggregation, and membrane integrity.

Forms Used

Capsules, tablets, powder

Dosage

100 to 2,000 milligrams a day

T=Therapeutic   **P**=Preventive   **B**=Both

Useful Combinations

Taurine may increase the effects of non-steroidal anti-inflammatory drugs (NSAIDs), such as aspirin. It is best taken with vitamin B_6.

Cautions

Do not use with high doses of alanine.

Signs of Overdose

None known

Food Sources

Meats, seafood, poultry

Use

Disorder	T	P	B
Abnormal heartbeat	✓		
Alcoholism	✓		
Angina	✓		
Cardiomyopathy	✓		
Cirrhosis	✓		
Congestive heart failure	✓		
Diabetes	✓		
Heart attack	✓		
High blood pressure	✓		
Palpitations	✓		
Seizures	✓		

▶ THREONINE

Abbreviation

Thr

Other Name

L-threonine

Description

Threonine is an essential amino acid, which means it is not synthesized by the body and therefore must be provided by the diet. Threonine is essential for the formation of collagen and elastin. It is present in the heart, central nervous system, and skeletal muscles.

Forms Used

Capsules, tablets, powder

Dosage

1,000 to 2,000 milligrams a day

Useful Combinations

It may be beneficial to take threonine when taking vitamin B_6 or antiepileptic medications.

Cautions

None known

Signs of Overdose

None known

Food Sources

Seafood, turkey, chicken, pork, beef, kidney beans, peas, peanuts, eggs

Use

Disorder	T	P	B
Leg ulcers	✓		
Lou Gehrig's disease	✓		
Seizures	✓		
Spastic paralysis	✓		

▶ TRYPTOPHAN

Abbreviation

Trp

Other Names

Tryptophane, L-tryptophan

Description

Tryptophan is an essential amino acid, which means it is not synthesized by the body and therefore must be provided by the diet. It is a precursor to the neurotransmitter serotonin and the B vitamin niacin. Serotonin has been shown to improve sleep and mood, control pain, and decrease inflammation.

Forms Used

Capsules, tablets

Dosage

1,000 to 2,000 milligrams a day

Useful Combinations

Tryptophan works together with vitamin B_6. Niacin and possibly niacinamide increase synthesis of tryptophan.

T=Therapeutic **P**=Preventive **B**=Both

Cautions

Currently, tryptophan is available only by prescription and should not be used without consulting a physician. Tryptophan should not be used with monoamine oxidase (MAO) inhibitors or antidepressants.

Signs of Overdose

Muscle pain, nausea, vomiting

Food Sources

Fish (especially dried), turkey, chicken, beef, eggs, peanuts, soybeans (but not other beans), pumpkin seeds, sunflower seeds

Use

Disorder	T	P	B
Bipolar disorder		✓	
Depression	✓		
Down syndrome	✓		
Hartnup's disease	✓		
Headache	✓		
Insomnia	✓		
Pellagra	✓		
Schizophrenia	✓		

▶ TYROSINE

Abbreviation

Tyr

Other Name

L-tyrosine

Description

Tyrosine is an amino acid that increases the levels of neurotransmitters in the brain known as catecholamines, which include norepinephrine, epinephrine, L-dopa, and dopamine. Tyrosine has been shown to be beneficial in patients with Parkinson's disease, which is characterized by a deficiency of dopamine. Tyrosine may also be beneficial in individuals with depression because it increases norepinephrine levels, which are often low in individuals with depression. Because thyroid hormones are made from tyrosine, individuals with an underactive thyroid gland may also benefit from tyrosine supplementation.

Forms Used

Capsules, tablets, powder

Dosage

500 to 2,000 milligrams a day

Useful Combinations

Useful combinations to be taken along with tyrosine include copper, folic acid, S-adenosylmethionine (SAM), and vitamin B_6.

Cautions

Do not use with high doses of phenylalanine. Do not take with monoamine oxidase (MAO) inhibitors and antidepressants. Tyrosine should be avoided by individuals with schizophrenia.

Signs of Overdose

Diarrhea, nausea, vomiting, nervousness

Food Sources

Seafood, turkey, chicken, pork, beef, eggs, beans, grains, nuts, sesame seeds, sunflower seeds

Use

Disorder	T	P	B
Alzheimer's disease	✓		
Autoimmune thyroiditis	✓		
Depression	✓		
Goiter	✓		
L-dopa therapy	✓		
Narcolepsy	✓		
Parkinson's disease	✓		
Phenylketonuria	✓		
Renal failure	✓		
Stress			✓
Underactive thyroid	✓		

T=Therapeutic　P=Preventive　B=Both

▶ VALINE

Abbreviation

Val

Other Name

L-valine

Description

Valine is a branched-chain amino acid that enhances muscle recovery after physical stress. It works together with other branched-chain amino acids, such as leucine and isoleucine.

Forms Used

Capsules, tablets, powder

Dosage

600 to 2,000 milligrams a day

Useful Combinations

Useful combinations include magnesium and vitamin B_6.

Cautions

Do not use tryptophan while taking valine. Individuals with kidney or liver disease should not take high dosages of amino acids.

Signs of Overdose

None known

Food Sources

Chicken, beef, seafood, turkey, nuts, seeds

Use

Disorder	T	P	B
Exercise endurance	✓		
Lou Gehrig's disease	✓		
Stress	✓		
Surgery recovery	✓		

▶ VANADIUM

Abbreviation

V

Other Name

Vanadyl sulfate

Description

Vanadium has been shown to improve blood sugar metabolism in individuals with diabetes. Vanadium may improve mineralization of bones and teeth and may also improve glucose tolerance.

Forms Used

Capsules, tablets

Dosage

20 to 100 micrograms a day

Useful Combinations

Vanadium may be synergistic with chromium.

Cautions

Do not use high doses and do not combine with monoamine oxidase (MAO) inhibitor antidepressants. High levels of vanadium in individuals have been linked to manic-depressive states.

Signs of Overdose

High blood pressure, cramps, diarrhea

Food Sources

Buckwheat, parsley, soybeans, eggs, sunflower seed oil, oats, olive oil, sunflower seeds, corn, green beans, peanut oil, carrots, cabbage, garlic, seafood

Use

Disorder	T	P	B
Depression	✓		
Diabetes	✓		

▶ VITAMIN A (RETINOL)

Abbreviation

Vit A

Other Name

Retinol

T=Therapeutic   **P**=Preventive   **B**=Both

THE PATIENT FILE

An A⁺ Anti-Acne Approach

Severe acne dotted Susan's cheeks, chin, and forehead. The pimples embarrassed her so much that she shied away from social activities and did not even want to show her face in school.

Like many 15-year-olds, Susan ate a lot of nutritionally barren junk food. Potato chips, french fries, fast-food hamburgers, chocolate, cake, soda pop, and the like were the mainstays of her diet—and most likely the source of her dermatological problem.

That had to change. She had to eliminate all of the junk food from her diet and start eating a healthy salad for lunch or dinner with five different vegetables. I told her to eat three different fruits every day and to replace the soda with all-natural fresh fruit juice.

I also put her on a multivitamin, but her primary supplemental prescription was for 50,000 international units of skin-conditioning vitamin A twice a day. That's an enormous dosage, far more than many people require, but Susan's problem demanded it. No one should take this amount except under a physician's direction.

With the prescription came a caution. Large amounts of vitamin A can cause fetal birth defects, among other side effects, and so I stressed to Susan the overriding need for her to practice safe sex and to insist that any partner use a condom.

A month later, I saw an almost entirely different face when Susan walked into my office. Most of the acne had vanished, save for a few blemishes on her cheeks. She was elated. She also felt better, more energetic, and more optimistic. And in the process of totally revamping her diet, she had found a new place to hang out with friends—a healthy eatery that features fresh juices and organic foods.

Susan told me that her period had started 2 days earlier. That, I thought, accounted for the remaining pimples. Because of hormonal surges that occur as menstruation nears, many women get acne flare-ups. I figured that the blemishes would disappear after her period ended, but for some added insurance, I told her to take 50 milligrams of vitamin B₆ each day for 6 months.

Curious about whether my hunch was correct, I called Susan 2 weeks later. Sure enough, the lingering acne had gone away with her period.

Description

Vitamin A is a fat-soluble vitamin. There are several active forms of vitamin A, including retinol, retinoic acid, and retinyl esters. Beta-carotene is a precursor to vitamin A, meaning that some carotenes can be converted into vitamin A in the body. Vitamin A is needed to maintain normal vision, especially vision in dim or dark situations. Vitamin A is also required to build and maintain healthy skin and mucous membranes, and studies suggest that it may help prevent epithelial cell cancers such as cervical and colon cancers. In addition, vitamin A is essential for reproduction, the formation of bones and teeth, and proper immune function.

Forms Used

Capsules, tablets, liquid

T=Therapeutic   **P**=Preventive   **B**=Both

Dosage

5,000 to 25,000 international units a day. A typical dosage is 5,000 international units a day; individuals with cancer should take dosages at the higher end of the range.

Useful Combinations

Vitamin A works best when taken with vitamin E. Vitamin A may also be synergistic with zinc in promoting wound healing. Vitamin A may prevent some of the adverse effects of corticosteroids.

Cautions

High dosages of vitamin A may turn the skin a yellow-orange color. A common sign of vitamin A deficiency is night blindness. Vitamin A should be used in small amounts in individuals with liver disease. High dosages of vitamin A can cause liver damage. Do not use more than 5,000 international units a day of vitamin A if you are pregnant or have any chance of becoming pregnant, because high dosages of vitamin A can cause birth defects. Premenopausal women in general should avoid taking vitamin A in doses over 5,000 international units; use beta-carotene instead.

Signs of Overdose

Jaundice, high blood pressure, headache, soreness, fatigue, joint pain, muscle pain, dry skin

Food Sources

Liver, red chili peppers, dandelion greens, carrots, dried apricots, collard greens

Use

Disorder	T	P	B
Abscesses	✓		
Acne	✓		
Aging		✓	
Allergies	✓		
Bladder infection	✓		
Boils	✓		
Breast cancer		✓	

Disorder	T	P	B
Cancer			✓
Cataracts			✓
Celiac disease	✓		
Cervical dysplasia	✓		
Colds	✓		
Colorectal cancer		✓	
Congestive heart failure	✓		
Conjunctivitis	✓		
Contact dermatitis	✓		
Coronary heart disease	✓		
Coughs	✓		
Crohn's disease	✓		
Dandruff	✓		
Down syndrome	✓		
Dry eyes	✓		
Dry skin	✓		
Eczema	✓		
Emphysema	✓		
Fever	✓		
Gastritis	✓		
Glaucoma	✓		
Gum disease			✓
Heart attack	✓		
High blood pressure	✓		
High cholesterol levels		✓	
HIV infection and AIDS	✓		
Immunodeficiency	✓		
Influenza	✓		
Intestinal atrophy	✓		
Leg ulcers	✓		
Leukoplakia	✓		
Lung cancer	✓		
Lupus	✓		
Macular degeneration			✓
Measles and rubella		✓	
Menopausal symptoms		✓	
Menstrual bleeding (excessive)	✓		
Mononucleosis	✓		
Mumps	✓		
Night blindness			✓
Overactive thyroid		✓	
Parkinson's disease			✓
Peptic ulcer			✓
Periodontal disease	✓		
Psoriasis	✓		
Rosacea	✓		
Skin cancer	✓		
Stomach cancer	✓		
Surgery recovery		✓	
Ulcerative colitis		✓	
Underactive thyroid	✓		
Vaginitis	✓		
Viral infection		✓	
Wounds	✓		

T=Therapeutic   **P**=Preventive   **B**=Both

▶ VITAMIN B$_1$ (THIAMIN)[1]

Abbreviation

B$_1$

Other Names

Thiamin, thiamine

Description

Vitamin B$_1$ is essential for converting carbohydrates into energy and fat. It also functions as a coenzyme to produce acetylcholine, which is needed for proper nervous system functioning. Vitamin B$_1$ deficiency is common in alcoholics, causing Wernicke-Korsakoff syndrome, which is characterized by uncoordinated movements (ataxia) and the inability to remember recent events. Vitamin B$_1$ deficiency can also affect the outer or peripheral nerves, causing leg cramps, numbness, partial paralysis of the toes, and a burning sensation in the feet that gets worse at night. Severe thiamin deficiency also causes a syndrome called beriberi, which includes such symptoms as mental confusion, muscle wasting, fluid retention, high blood pressure, difficulty walking, and heart disturbances. The need for vitamin B$_1$ is dependent upon energy expenditure; therefore, athletes have higher requirements than sedentary individuals.

Forms Used

Capsules, tablets, liquid

Dosage

10 to 50 milligrams a day. A typical dosage is 10 to 25 milligrams a day; individuals with alcoholism or vitamin B$_1$–related illnesses should take dosages at the higher end of the range, from 50 to 100 milligrams a day.

Useful Combinations

Vitamin B$_1$ is synergistic with magnesium and vitamins B$_6$ and B$_{12}$.

Cautions

Alcohol and phenytoin (Dilantin) may inhibit thiamin absorption.

Signs of Overdose

None known

Food Sources

Brewer's yeast, wheat germ, sunflower seeds, pine nuts, peanuts, soybeans, Brazil nuts

Use

Disorder	T	P	B
Alcoholism	✓		
Attention deficit hyperactivity disorder	✓		
Canker sores	✓		
Cirrhosis	✓		
Depression	✓		
Diabetic neuropathy	✓		
Fibromyalgia	✓		
Neuralgia and neuritis	✓		

▶ VITAMIN B$_2$ (RIBOFLAVIN)

Abbreviation

B$_2$

Other Name

Riboflavin

Description

Vitamin B$_2$, or riboflavin, is important in energy production. It also helps maintain the skin, the mucous membranes, the cornea of the eye, and nerve function. A deficiency can cause the eyes to be overly sensitive to light and can also produce skin and mucous membrane disorders. Vitamin B$_2$ deficiency also may cause scaly, greasy, reddened skin or cracking of the skin around the nose, mouth, ears, and eyelids; it may cause the skin to have a rough-

T=Therapeutic   **P**=Preventive   **B**=Both

ened look and the tongue to have a magenta color, with the lips red and cracked; or it may cause anemia and seborrheic dermatitis. Riboflavin is the B vitamin that turns urine a yellow color.

Forms Used

Capsules, tablets, liquid

Dosage

10 to 100 milligrams a day

Useful Combinations

Riboflavin may offset side effects of phenothiazines and doxorubicin. Riboflavin may potentiate antidepressants.

Cautions

Antimalarial medications may interfere with riboflavin metabolism.

Signs of Overdose

None known

Food Sources

Brewer's yeast, liver, almonds, wheat germ, wild rice, mushrooms

Use

Disorder	T	P	B
Appetite loss	✓		
Attention deficit hyperactivity disorder	✓		
Canker sores	✓		
Carpal tunnel syndrome	✓		
Cataracts		✓	
Depression	✓		
Glossitis	✓		
Growth retardation	✓		
Hair thinning or loss		✓	
Headache	✓		
Leg cramps	✓		
Macular degeneration		✓	
Migraine		✓	
Rosacea	✓		
Sickle cell disease	✓		
Underactive thyroid	✓		
Weak fingernails	✓		

▶ VITAMIN B$_3$ (NIACIN)

See also Niacinamide

Abbreviation

B$_3$

Other Names

Niacin, nicotinic acid

Description

Vitamin B$_3$ (niacin) is essential for the breakdown of carbohydrates, protein, and fat, as well as the synthesis of fatty acids and steroids. Niacin deficiency causes a disease called pellagra, which includes symptoms such as fatigue, decreased appetite, indigestion, dermatitis, diarrhea, and dementia. Niacin deficiency has been associated with a predominantly corn diet. This is attributed to the low tryptophan content of corn and the fact that niacin is bound as niacinogen, a compound that is not well-absorbed. The treatment of corn with limewater, as is done in Mexico and Central and South America in the process of making tortillas, enhances the availability of niacin. As a result, people from these areas do not suffer from pellagra; however, pellagra is still common in India, China, and Africa.

Forms Used

Capsules, tablets

Dosage

Niacin: 10 to 50 milligrams a day; sustained-release niacin: 50 milligrams twice a day. A typical dosage of niacin is 10 to 35 milligrams a day; individuals with the diseases and conditions listed under "Use" below should take dosages at the higher end of the range but watch for side effects.

T=Therapeutic$\quad$**P**=Preventive$\quad$**B**=Both

Useful Combinations

Niacin works synergistically with chromium and B-complex vitamins. Niacin can be combined with a lipid-lowering drug to increase the drug's effect on lowering cholesterol and triglyceride levels.

Cautions

Do not take vitamin B₃ in high doses if you have gout, peptic ulcer, or diabetes. High doses can damage the liver. Sustained-release niacin is recommended to prevent liver damage. Individuals taking niacin in large doses (50 milligrams a day) should be monitored by a physician who tests their liver enzymes regularly.

Signs of Overdose

Nausea, skin rash, jaundice, elevated liver enzymes, flushing and itching of the skin, headaches, cramps, gastrointestinal irritation

Food Sources

Brewer's yeast, rice bran, wheat bran, peanuts, liver, turkey, chicken, trout, halibut

Use

Disorder	T	P	B
Alcoholism	✓		
Asthma	✓		
Attention deficit hyperactivity disorder	✓		
Bad breath	✓		
Cataracts	✓		
Glossitis	✓		
High cholesterol levels	✓		
Migraine	✓		
Pellagra	✓		
Raynaud's disease	✓		
Underactive thyroid	✓		

▶ VITAMIN B₅ (PANTOTHENIC ACID)

Abbreviation

B₅

Other Names

Pantothenic acid, pantothethine

Description

Vitamin B₅ is involved in the metabolism of fats, carbohydrates, and some amino acids and also helps regulate stress hormones such as adrenalin, which is produced by the adrenal glands. Vitamin B₅ deficiency is common in alcoholics and in individuals with severe malnutrition. Vitamin B₅ may promote wound healing and reduce the side effects of surgery.

Forms Used

Capsules, tablets

Dosage

5 to 50 milligrams a day. A typical dosage is 5 milligrams a day; individuals with high cholesterol and high blood lipids should take dosages at the higher end of the range.

Useful Combinations

Vitamin B₅ is best absorbed when combined with a B-complex vitamin.

Cautions

None known

Sign of Overdose

Diarrhea

Food Sources

Brewer's yeast, liver, kidney, peanuts, mushrooms, soybeans, split peas, perch, blue cheese

Use

Disorder	T	P	B
Adrenal insufficiency	✓		
Attention deficit hyperactivity disorder	✓		
High cholesterol levels	✓		
Intestinal atrophy	✓		
Obesity	✓		
Rheumatoid arthritis	✓		
Surgery recovery	✓		

T=Therapeutic   **P**=Preventive   **B**=Both

▶ VITAMIN B$_6$

Abbreviation

B$_6$

Other Names

Pyridoxine, pyridoxine-5-phosphate (P5P)

Description

Vitamin B$_6$ is involved in the metabolism of protein, carbohydrates, and fat. Without vitamin B$_6$, the nonessential amino acids cannot be synthesized. Vitamin B$_6$ is also needed for the synthesis of hemoglobin, which is the oxygen-carrying molecule in red blood cells, and the synthesis of white blood cells, which play an important role in the immune system. Vitamin B$_6$ is required for the conversion of tryptophan to niacin and for the synthesis of other neurotransmitters. Vitamin B$_6$ deficiency may cause depression, headaches, confusion, seizures, dermatitis, glucose intolerance, cracking of the lips, eczema, and anemia. Alcoholics are at a high risk for vitamin B$_6$ deficiency. Vitamin B$_6$ is beneficial for the treatment of "Chinese restaurant syndrome," or MSG (monosodium glutamate) sensitivity, which can cause flushing, headaches, and tingling sensations after a sensitive person eats Chinese food (or other food with high MSG content). Vitamin B$_6$ has also been shown to lower homocysteine levels, therefore lowering one's risk for coronary heart disease and stroke.

Forms Used

Capsules, tablets

Dosage

2 to 200 milligrams a day

Useful Combinations

Vitamin B$_6$ may offset the side effects of oral contraceptives, monoamine oxidase (MAO) inhibitors, isoniazid, and theophylline drugs. Vitamin B$_6$ works together with folic acid and vitamin B$_{12}$. It is also a cofactor in essential fatty acid metabolism. Magnesium and vitamin B$_2$ (riboflavin) enhance the absorption of vitamin B$_6$.

Cautions

Vitamin B$_6$ may reduce milk production in lactating women. Large doses of vitamin B$_6$ may increase the need for other B vitamins, essential fatty acids, magnesium, and zinc. Taking high doses of vitamin B$_6$ for extended periods of time may cause sensory neuropathy. Pregnant women should not take more than 100 milligrams a day. As many as 40 different drugs have been found to interfere with vitamin B$_6$ metabolism, including hydralazine (a high blood pressure drug), isoniazid (a tuberculosis drug), dopamine, penicillamine, and oral contraceptives.

Signs of Overdose

Tingling in hands and feet, insomnia, anxiety

Food Sources

Brewer's yeast, sunflower seeds, wheat germ, tuna, liver, soybeans, walnuts, salmon

Use

Disorder	T	P	B
Acne	✓		
Alcoholism	✓		
Asthma		✓	
Attention deficit hyperactivity disorder	✓		
Autism	✓		
Breast tenderness	✓		
Canker sores	✓		
Carpal tunnel syndrome	✓		
Cirrhosis	✓		
Coronary heart disease		✓	
Crohn's disease	✓		
Depression	✓		
Diabetes		✓	
Diabetic neuropathy	✓		
Fibrocystic breasts	✓		

T=Therapeutic **P**=Preventive **B**=Both

Disorder	T	P	B
Glossitis	✓		
Hair thinning or loss	✓		
Hepatitis	✓		
Intermittent claudication	✓		
Isoniazid drug therapy		✓	
Kidney stones		✓	
Lou Gehrig's disease	✓		
Low blood sugar	✓		
Menopausal symptoms		✓	
Menstrual cramps	✓		
Monosodium glutamate intolerance		✓	
Morning sickness	✓		
Multiple sclerosis	✓		
Myasthenia gravis	✓		
Osteoporosis		✓	
Parkinson's disease	✓		
Pregnancy complications		✓	
Premenstrual acne	✓		
Premenstrual syndrome	✓		
Renal failure	✓		
Seizures	✓		
Stroke	✓		
Theophylline drug therapy		✓	

▶ VITAMIN B$_{12}$

Abbreviation

B$_{12}$

Other Names

Cobalamin, hydroxycobalamin, methylcobalamin

Description

Vitamin B$_{12}$ is needed to make blood cells and nerve sheaths for proper nerve function. It is also needed for normal fatty acid and DNA synthesis. A vitamin B$_{12}$ deficiency can produce pernicious (mcgaloblastic) anemia. Individuals most at risk in developing a B$_{12}$ deficiency are strict vegetarians who eat no animal products and those individuals who are unable to absorb B$_{12}$ from food. The earliest warning signs of vitamin B$_{12}$ deficiency are fatigue and numbness, "pins and needles" sensations, and burning feelings, all of which may indicate nerve damage.

Forms Used

Tablets, liquid, injection

Dosage

1,000 micrograms a day

Useful Combinations

Vitamin B$_{12}$ works together with folic acid and vitamin B$_6$. Vitamin B$_{12}$ may prevent side effects of beta blocker drugs and oral hypoglycemic drugs, and it works synergistically with insulin. Vitamin B$_{12}$ may improve melatonin secretion.

Cautions

People with acne should use vitamin B$_{12}$ with caution because it can make the condition worse. Vitamin B$_{12}$ absorption may be impaired by histamine-2 blockers, potassium citrate, potassium chloride, and oral hypoglycemic agents. Large doses of vitamin B$_{12}$ may increase the requirement for folic acid. AZT (azicothymidine) may cause deficiencies of folic acid and vitamins B$_{12}$ and E.

Sign of Overdose

Acne

Food Sources

Liver, clams, oysters, sardines, egg yolks, trout, salmon, tuna, lamb, cheese

Use

Disorder	T	P	B
Aging (loss of strength)	✓		
Alzheimer's disease			✓
Anxiety attacks	✓		
Asthma		✓	
Attention deficit hyperactivity disorder	✓		
Bell's palsy	✓		
Bipolar disorder		✓	
Canker sores	✓		
Cervical dysplasia	✓		
Coronary heart disease		✓	
Cradle cap	✓		
Crohn's disease	✓		
Dandruff	✓		
Depression		✓	

T=Therapeutic   **P**=Preventive   **B**=Both

Disorder	T	P	B
Diabetic neuropathy	✓		
Dry skin	✓		
Fatigue	✓		
Hepatitis	✓		
Hives	✓		
Leg cramps	✓		
Low blood sugar	✓		
Lupus		✓	
Male infertility	✓		
Megaloblastic anemia			✓
Multiple sclerosis	✓		
Neuralgia and neuritis	✓		
Osteoporosis	✓		
Pernicious anemia	✓		
Rosacea	✓		
Schizophrenia	✓		
Shingles	✓		
Stroke	✓		
Tinnitus	✓		
Vitiligo	✓		

▶ VITAMIN C

Abbreviation

Vit C

Other Names

Ascorbate, ascorbic acid

Description

Vitamin C is essential for the synthesis of collagen, the basis of all connective tissue in the body. The absence of such synthesis results in a disease called scurvy, which causes poor wound healing, bone and joint pain, bone fractures, improperly formed teeth, and bleeding. Vitamin C is also needed for the synthesis of neurotransmitters, thyroid and steroid hormones, bile acids, and DNA. Vitamin C is often depleted in smokers.

Forms Used

Tablets, liquid

Dosage

200 to 3,000 milligrams a day. A typical preventive dosage is 200 to 500 milligrams per day;

higher doses may be recommended for individuals with allergies as a natural anti-inflammatory.

Useful Combinations

Vitamin C enhances iron and copper absorption and is synergistic with aspirin.

Cautions

Do not abruptly stop taking high doses of vitamin C because doing so can cause stomach upset. Do not take vitamin C if you have renal disease or any of the following genetic disorders: glucose-6-phosphate dehydrogenase deficiency, genetic oxalate metabolism defects, hemochromatosis. Doses over 250 milligrams of vitamin C interfere with stool occult blood testing. High doses of vitamin C can cause diarrhea in some individuals.

Signs of Overdose

Diarrhea, gas, abdominal pain

Food Sources

Red chili peppers, guavas, red sweet peppers, kale greens, collard greens, green peppers, broccoli, orange juice

Use

Disorder	T	P	B
Abscesses	✓		
Acne	✓		
Aging		✓	
Allergies	✓		
Alzheimer's disease		✓	
Aspirin therapy	✓		
Asthma	✓		
Autoimmune disease		✓	
Bipolar disorder		✓	
Bladder infection	✓		
Boils	✓		
Breast cancer		✓	
Bruises	✓		
Cancer			✓
Capillary fragility	✓		
Cardiomyopathy	✓		
Cataracts	✓		
Cervical dysplasia	✓		
Chronic pain	✓		
Colds	✓		

T=Therapeutic   **P**=Preventive   **B**=Both

Disorder	T	P	B
Colorectal cancer		✓	
Congestive heart failure	✓		
Conjunctivitis	✓		
Contact dermatitis	✓		
Coronary heart disease	✓		
Coughs	✓		
Crohn's disease	✓		
Dandruff	✓		
Depression		✓	
Diabetes			✓
Disk problems	✓		
Down syndrome	✓		
Dry skin	✓		
Ear infection	✓		
Eczema	✓		
Emphysema	✓		
Fever	✓		
Glaucoma	✓		
Gout	✓		
Gum disease	✓		
Hair thinning or loss		✓	
Hay fever	✓		
Heart attack	✓		
Heavy metal toxicity	✓		
Hepatitis	✓		
Hereditary angioedema	✓		
High blood pressure	✓		
High cholesterol levels		✓	
Hives	✓		
HIV infection and AIDS	✓		
Hot flashes			✓
Immunodeficiency	✓		
Inflammation	✓		
Influenza	✓		
Intermittent claudication	✓		
Iron-deficiency anemia	✓		
Joint pain	✓		
Kidney stones		✓	
Laryngitis	✓		
Leg ulcers	✓		
Low blood sugar	✓		
Lung cancer	✓		
Lupus	✓		
Lymph node swelling	✓		
Macular degeneration	✓		
Male infertility	✓		
Measles and rubella		✓	
Menopausal symptoms		✓	
Menstrual bleeding (excessive)		✓	
Mononucleosis	✓		
Morning sickness	✓		
Multiple sclerosis	✓		
Mumps		✓	
Overactive thyroid		✓	

Disorder	T	P	B
Parkinson's disease	✓		
Peptic ulcer			✓
Periodontal disease	✓		
Rosacea	✓		
Schizophrenia	✓		
Scurvy	✓		
Shingles	✓		
Sinusitis	✓		
Skin cancer		✓	
Sore throat	✓		
Stomach cancer	✓		
Sunburn	✓		
Surgery recovery		✓	
Ulcerative colitis		✓	
Vaginitis	✓		
Varicose veins	✓		
Venous insufficiency	✓		
Viral infection		✓	
Vitiligo	✓		
Wounds		✓	

▶ VITAMIN D

Abbreviation

Vit D

Other Name

Cholecalciferol

Description

Vitamin D is a fat-soluble vitamin that is often called the sunshine vitamin because 10 to 15 minutes of sun exposure three times a week will provide the daily requirement. Vitamin D helps build and maintain teeth and bones and is required for the body to absorb and metabolize calcium and phosphorus. Children who do not get enough vitamin D may develop rickets, other skeletal deformities, and malformed teeth. Adults with vitamin D deficiency may develop osteomalacia (bone softening), muscle twitching, cramps, and convulsions.

Forms Used

Capsules, tablets

T=Therapeutic　**P**=Preventive　**B**=Both

THE PATIENT FILE

Supplements Support Dietary Decisions

The interactions between what we eat and what we experience often are fraught with nuance and the unknown. Supplements can offer insurance and assurance.

When Karen, a 32-year-old woman, came to me complaining of recurring canker sores in her mouth, I figured that she had either a food sensitivity or a nutrient deficiency—or that she was under a tremendous amount of stress. I talked to Karen about reducing the stress in her life. I prescribed a good multiple vitamin containing folic acid, iron, vitamin B$_{12}$, and zinc, nutrients that have been associated with alleviating recurrent canker sores. I also put her on a diet that contained no gluten, another culprit in the appearance of those tiny but painful mouth ulcers.

A no-gluten diet means eating foods that contain no wheat, rye, barley, or oats. I also recommended more bioflavonoid-rich foods such as blueberries, cherries, raspberries, plums, grapes, and other fruits.

A month later, Karen returned to my office free from canker sores. As an experiment to see what had actually caused them, I told her to resume eating foods, such as bread, that contain wheat.

The canker sores reappeared almost immediately.

Back off the wheat, I told her, convinced that she was allergic to it. I prescribed that she refrain from eating wheat products for the next 3 months.

Two months later, she had no canker sores. I told her to live wheat-free for another month and return for a follow-up visit. Yes, frequent checkups are inconvenient, but they're absolutely necessary to gauge how a patient is faring.

When Karen returned 30 days later, still free of canker sores, I told her to start eating bread, cereal, and other wheat products—but no more than three times a week. Many people suffer the consequences of such food sensitivity. But if you take a sabbatical from the foods that bother you, then eat them only occasionally, at most three times a week, chances are you'll be just fine.

Ask Karen. For the past 3 years, she hasn't had a single canker sore.

Dosage

200 to 400 international units a day, up to 600 IU aged 70 and older

Useful Combinations

Vitamin D may prevent some of the side effects of anticonvulsants and corticosteroids. It also may increase the absorption of calcium.

Cautions

Vitamin D can be toxic in high doses. Too much vitamin D can lead to kidney damage or to calcification of the heart and other soft tissues. Therefore, supplementation of vitamin D is not necessary in individuals who have high levels of sun exposure. Prednisone interferes with the conversion of vitamin D to its biologically active form. Anticonvulsants may cause deficiencies of folic acid and vitamin D. Individuals with sarcoidosis or hyperparathyroidism should not supplement with vitamin D.

Signs of Overdose

Elevated calcium levels in the blood, diarrhea, headache

T=Therapeutic   **P**=Preventive   **B**=Both

Food Sources

Sardines, herring, butter, liver, egg yolks, fortified milk, fortified cereals

Use

Disorder	T	P	B
Breast cancer			✓
Celiac disease	✓		
Cirrhosis	✓		
Contact dermatitis	✓		
Crohn's disease	✓		
Fractured bone	✓		
Osteoporosis			✓
Psoriasis	✓		
Seizures	✓		
Weak fingernails	✓		

▶ VITAMIN E

Abbreviation

Vit E

Other Names

Alpha-tocopherol, d-alpha-tocopherol (natural form), dl-alpha-tocopherol (synthetic form)

Description

Vitamin E is a fat-soluble vitamin that acts as an antioxidant. It prevents oxidation of vitamin A and polyunsaturated fatty acids, thus helping to maintain cell membranes (including those of red blood cells). Vitamin E also protects the immune system from damage during times of oxidative stress. Thus, vitamin E can help prevent coronary heart disease and stroke. Vitamin E deficiency may cause nerve damage, muscle weakness, poor coordination, involuntary movement of the eyes, and hemolytic anemia.

Forms Used

Capsules, liquid

Dosage

400 to 800 international units a day; apply topically to scar tissue and to skin for skin cancer

Useful Combinations

Vitamin E may offset the side effects of the pharmaceuticals griseofulvin, AZT (azidothymidine), and phenothiazines. Supplementation with vitamin E reduces the toxicity of AZT and increases its efficacy, allowing a reduction in dosage. Vitamin E prevents oxidation of essential fatty acids. Vitamin E improves the absorption of vitamins A and B_{12}.

Cautions

On rare occasions, vitamin E may raise blood pressure. Vitamin E inhibits iron absorption. Large doses of vitamin E may increase the effects of warfarin and promote bleeding; do not take large doses without physician supervision. Vitamin E may thin the blood. Cigarettes may deplete vitamin C, vitamin E, carotenoids, and vitamin A. AZT may cause deficiencies of folic acid and vitamins B_{12} and E.

Sign of Overdose

High blood pressure

Food Sources

Wheat germ oil, sunflower seeds and oil, safflower oil, almonds, sesame oil

Use

Disorder	T	P	B
Abnormal heartbeat	✓		
Abscesses	✓		
Acne	✓		
Aging		✓	
Alcoholism	✓		
Alzheimer's disease			✓
Angina			✓
Autoimmune disease		✓	
Breast cancer		✓	
Breast tenderness	✓		
Bruises		✓	
Burns			✓
Cancer		✓	
Capillary fragility	✓		
Cardiomyopathy	✓		
Cataracts			✓
Celiac disease	✓		
Cervical dysplasia	✓		
Chondromalacia	✓		
Cirrhosis	✓		

T=Therapeutic   **P**=Preventive   **B**=Both

Disorder	T	P	B
Colorectal cancer		✓	
Congestive heart failure	✓		
Contact dermatitis	✓		
Coronary heart disease	✓		
Crohn's disease	✓		
Cuts and scrapes	✓		
Dandruff	✓		
Diabetes	✓		
Diabetic neuropathy	✓		
Down syndrome	✓		
Dry skin	✓		
Dupuytren's contracture	✓		
Eczema	✓		
Emphysema	✓		
Enlarged scars	✓		
Fibrocystic breasts	✓		
Gastritis	✓		
Glaucoma	✓		
Hair thinning or loss		✓	
Heart attack	✓		
Herpes simplex	✓		
High blood pressure	✓		
High cholesterol levels			✓
HIV infection and AIDS	✓		
Hot flashes	✓		
Immunodeficiency	✓		
Impotence	✓		
Intermittent claudication			✓
Leg cramps	✓		
Leg ulcers	✓		
Lou Gehrig's disease	✓		
Lung cancer	✓		
Lupus		✓	
Lymph node swelling	✓		
Male infertility	✓		
Menopausal symptoms		✓	
Menstrual bleeding (excessive)	✓		
Multiple sclerosis	✓		
Muscular dystrophy	✓		
Neuralgia and neuritis	✓		
Osgood-Schlatter disease	✓		
Osteoarthritis	✓		
Overactive thyroid		✓	
Palpitations	✓		
Parkinson's disease	✓		
Peptic ulcer	✓		
Periodontal disease	✓		
Peyronie's disease		✓	
Premenstrual syndrome	✓		
Psoriasis		✓	
Raynaud's disease	✓		
Restless legs syndrome	✓		
Rosacea	✓		
Scleroderma	✓		

Disorder	T	P	B
Seizures	✓		
Shingles	✓		
Skin cancer	✓		
Stomach cancer	✓		
Stroke			✓
Sunburn	✓		
Surgery recovery			✓
Tardive dyskinesia	✓		
Ulcerative colitis			✓
Varicose veins			✓
Venous insufficiency	✓		
Wounds			✓

▶ VITAMIN K

Abbreviation

Vit K

Other Name

Phylloquinone

Description

Vitamin K is a fat-soluble vitamin that is involved in blood clotting (coagulation). Vitamin K is needed for the production of the blood protein prothrombin and other blood-clotting factors that are needed to produce fibrin, a protein that forms the structure of a blood clot. Vitamin K also works with vitamin D in regulating blood calcium levels and may play a role in depositing minerals in bone.

Forms Used

Capsules, tablets, injection

Dosage

50 to 80 micrograms a day

Useful Combinations

Vitamin K may enhance calcium absorption.

Cautions

Unmonitored use during warfarin therapy can reduce the drug's efficacy. Vitamin K may interfere with blood-thinner medications. Vitamin K deficiency often results from long-term use of antibiotics.

T=Therapeutic   **P**=Preventive   **B**=Both

REMEDY	GENERAL CHARACTERISTICS	SPECIFIC SYMPTOMS	AGG & ALEV CONDITIONS
HAMAMELIS	Weakness • Exhaustion	Bloody nose • Hemorrhoids • Veins are dilated and fragile • Bleed easily • Veins are bruised, purple • Varicose veins are large, sore, and easily irritated	< during pregnancy • < during menstruation
LACHESIS	Jealousness • Envy, suspicion, anger • Sarcastic	Varicose veins with pink or black color • Varicose veins with full, bursting appearance	< during sleep • < upon waking • < touch • < pressure • < menopause or pregnancy • < before menstrual period • < heat
PULSATILLA	Sweet, affectionate • Weepy, clingy • Changeable moods	Restlessness • Redness and swelling • Tearing, stinging, sharp, intense pain • Pain changes location	< during pregnancy • > cold

▶ WOUNDS

REMEDY	GENERAL CHARACTERISTICS	SPECIFIC SYMPTOMS	AGG & ALEV CONDITIONS
APIS MELLIFICA	Swelling and edema of the injured area • The injured area is bright red	Puncture wounds • Feels hot • Stinging • Intense swelling	> cold
HEPAR SULPHURIS	Oversensitivity to pain • Anxiety • Irritability	Reddening with infection • Abscesses • Extreme pain • Skin heals slowly • Skin ulcers	< cold
HYPERICUM	Sadness • Nervous depression following a wound	Deep wound • Severe or shooting pain • Wounds to the fingers, toes, teeth, spine • Numbness and tingling on or near wound area • Injuries to large nerves • Contusions, lacerations, or puncture wounds	< touch
LEDUM	Dissatisfied	Puncture wounds • Bites and stings from insects • Cat bite • Steps on nail • Injured area feels cold to touch	> cold • > bathing
SILICEA	Yielding, refined, delicate individuals	Splinter still in wound • Abscesses anywhere on body • May help to promote expulsion of foreign bodies through the skin • Unhealthy skin where every wound becomes infected	< cold air

< worse with   > better with

Section B

Homeopathy by Remedy

▶ ACONITUM NAPELLUS

Description

Aconite, *Aconitum napellus*, is a plant found in mountainous areas of central and southern Europe, Russia, Scandinavia, and Central America. The whole plant is used to make the remedy.

Dosage

Three or four 30C pellets every 2 to 3 hours until symptoms improve. If there is no improvement after three doses, it is the wrong remedy. Lower doses may also be taken (6C, 6X, 12C, 12X). (The correct homeopathic remedy will work in any potency.) Lower dosages such as 6C or 6X may need to be repeated more often, as frequently as six times a day.

Use

ASTHMA

General Characteristics

One cheek red, the other pale

Specific Symptoms

Symptoms follow fright

Sudden onset

Restlessness

Anxiety

Fear of death

Agg & Alev Conditions

< after midnight

BLADDER INFECTION

Aconitum napellus is recommended within the first 24 hours of the onset of a bladder infection.

General Characteristics

Restlessness

Anxiety

Specific Symptoms

Infection follows chill or fright

Sudden onset of infection

Pressing pain

Agg & Alev Conditions

< night

BLEEDING

General Characteristics

Tremendous fear of death

Great thirst for cold drinks

Panic attacks

Specific Symptoms

Bright red blood

Restlessness

Anxiety

Shock and fear immediately after an injury or accident

Agg & Alev Conditions

< cold, dry wind

COLDS

Aconitum napellus is recommended within the first 24 hours of the onset of a cold,

< worse with   > better with

especially when the cold comes on suddenly.

General Characteristics

Thirst for cold drinks

Anxiety

Restlessness at night

Specific Symptoms

Sudden onset of a cold

High fever brought on by cold, dry wind

Sneezing

Burning sensation in throat

Pharyngitis

Tonsillitis

Agg & Alev Conditions

< cold, dry wind

> sleep

> open air

COUGHS

General Characteristics

Anxiety

Specific Symptoms

Brought on by exposure to cold, dry air

Short, dry, croupy, barking cough

Red, burning sensation in the tonsils

Bitter taste in mouth

Agg & Alev Conditions

< warm room

EAR INFECTION

General Characteristics

Anxiety

Restlessness

Specific Symptoms

Sudden onset of earache

Comes on after chill

Ear is red, hot, and painful

High fever

Agg & Alev Conditions

> warm applications

EYE INJURY

General Characteristics

Anxiety

Restlessness

Specific Symptoms

Foreign body in eye

Swollen, red, burning eyelid

Pain of scratched cornea following foreign-body removal

Photophobia

Agg & Alev Conditions

< light

< night

HEADACHE

General Characteristics

Restlessness

Anxiety

Thirst

Specific Symptoms

Following shock or exposure to wind

Sudden onset; violent, bursting

Band of pressure all around head or forehead

Throbbing in temples

Agg & Alev Conditions

< evening

< night

< getting up from bed

> open air

HEAT EXHAUSTION

General Characteristics

Restlessness

Complaints begin after fright or a sudden, shocking event

Specific Symptoms

Thirst

Anxiety

Red, dry throat

Headache from the heat

< worse with   > better with

Sudden onset of heat exhaustion

Complaints about very hot weather

Shock and fear immediately after episode of heat exhaustion

Agg & Alev Conditions

< cold wind

HEATSTROKE

General Characteristics

Restlessness

Thirst for cold drinks

Specific Symptoms

Anxiety

Physical and emotional restlessness

Sudden onset of heatstroke

Complaints about very hot weather

Hot, dry, swollen eyes

One cheek red, the other pale

Agg & Alev Conditions

< cold, dry wind

> open air

INFLUENZA

General Characteristics

Anxiety

Specific Symptoms

Brought on by cold, dry wind

Red, dry skin

Red, swollen tonsils

Burning sensation in throat

High fever

Thirst for cold water

Agg & Alev Conditions

< cold, dry wind

< heat

MEASLES AND RUBELLA

Aconitum napellus is recommended within the first 24 hours of the onset of measles.

General Characteristics

Restlessness

Anxiety

Specific Symptoms

Sudden onset of measles

Photophobia

Eye and nasal discharge

Hard, croupy cough

Flushed face

High fever

Thirst

Rash that itches and burns

Agg & Alev Conditions

< evening/night

< after midnight

< chill

> open air

> rest

MUMPS

Aconitum napellus is recommended within the first 24 hours of the onset of mumps.

General Characteristics

Restlessness

Panic

Fear of death

Specific Symptoms

Sudden onset of mumps

Flushes of heat in the face

Fever

Thirst

Bitter taste in mouth

Agg & Alev Conditions

< warmth

> open air

SORE THROAT

Aconitum napellus is recommended within the first 24 hours of the onset of a sore throat.

General Characteristics

Anxiety

Specific Symptoms

Sudden onset of sore throat

Follows exposure to cold

< worse with   > better with

High fever

Thirst

Agg & Alev Conditions

< night

< cold, dry wind

▶ ALLIUM CEPA

Description

Allium cepa is the common red onion. The whole onion is used to make the remedy.

Dosage

Three or four 30C pellets every 2 to 3 hours until symptoms improve. If there is no improvement after three doses, it is the wrong remedy. Lower doses may also be taken (6C, 6X, 12C, 12X).

Use

COLDS

General Characteristics

Eyes and nose run as if individual were peeling an onion

Rawness in the throat

Desire for onion

Specific Symptoms

Clear, watery discharge from eye; discharge is not irritating

Watery nasal discharge drips continuously

Acrid/burning discharge from nose

Throat pain from coughing

Tickling feeling in the throat

Agg & Alev Conditions

< warm room

> open air

HAY FEVER

General Characteristics

Desire for onion

Specific Symptoms

Clear or watery discharge from eye; discharge is not irritating

Acrid discharge from nose

Loss of smell

Profuse watery discharge from the nose

Agg & Alev Conditions

< flowers

< warm room

< on the left side

< late afternoon or evening

> open air

▶ AMBRA GRISEA

Description

Ambra grisea is a product of the sperm whale.

Dosage

Three or four 30C pellets every 2 to 3 hours until symptoms improve. If there is no improvement after three doses, it is the wrong remedy. Lower doses may also be taken (6C, 6X, 12C, 12X).

Use

ASTHMA

General Characteristics

Follows embarrassment, failure

Shyness

Specific Symptoms

Cough triggered by hearing music

Cough made worse by talking or reading out loud

Dry, nervous, spasmodic cough

Agg & Alev Conditions

< slight exertion

< music

> face down, knees to chest

< worse with   > better with

▶ ANTIMONIUM CRUDUM

Description

Antimonium crudum is produced from the mineral sulphide of antimony.

Dosage

Three or four 30C pellets every 2 to 3 hours until symptoms improve. If there is no improvement after three doses, it is the wrong remedy. Lower doses may also be taken (6C, 6X, 12C, 12X).

Use

CHICKENPOX

General Characteristics

Dislikes being touched, bathed, or looked at

Irritability

Specific Symptoms

Scaly rash that burns and itches

Cough

White tongue

Shooting pain if eruptions touched

Sores have a honeylike discharge

Agg & Alev Conditions

< heat

< cold bathing

< evening

> open air

> resting

INDIGESTION

General Characteristics

Lack of thirst

Craving for pickles

Loves food and eating

Specific Symptoms

Comes on after overeating

Belching

Thick white coating on tongue

Gets indigestion easily

Diarrhea from sour food, vinegar, and bread

Alternating diarrhea and constipation

Agg & Alev Conditions

> vomiting

NAUSEA/MOTION SICKNESS

General Characteristics

Lack of thirst

Irritability

Specific Symptoms

Comes on after eating starchy or acidic food or after overeating

White coating on tongue

Agg & Alev Conditions

< immediately after eating or drinking

< during a headache

▶ ANTIMONIUM TARTARICUM

Description

Antimonium tartaricum is a tartrate of the minerals antimony and potash.

Dosage

Three or four 30C pellets every 2 to 3 hours until symptoms improve. If there is no improvement after three doses, it is the wrong remedy. Lower doses may also be taken (6C, 6X, 12C, 12X).

Use

ASTHMA

General Characteristics

Drowsiness

Paleness

Specific Symptoms

Coarse, rattling respiration

Cannot get the mucus out

Lips may turn blue

< worse with   > better with

Agg & Alev Conditions

< cold

< damp

< 3:00 to 4:00 A.M.

> burping

> open air

CHICKENPOX

General Characteristics

Irritability

Whininess

Specific Symptoms

Rash that is slow to appear, then becomes
large pustules

Sores that leave a bluish red mark

Coughing

Sweating

Drowsiness

White coating on tongue

Agg & Alev Conditions

< evening

< damp cold

< warmth

> sitting up

COLDS

General Characteristics

Irritability

Overwhelming sleepiness during a cough
or bronchitis

Specific Symptoms

Rattling respiration

Lips may turn blue

Nausea and vomiting with a cough

Weakness

Drowsiness

Sweaty, pale face

Gasping

Nostrils flare with breathing

Coughs and bronchitis in the elderly, especially in the winter months

Agg & Alev Conditions

< lying down

< evening

> sitting up

COUGHS

General Characteristics

Lack of thirst

Overwhelming sleepiness during a cough
or bronchitis

Specific Symptoms

Worsening cough

Pale face

Exhaustion

Weakness that prevents patient from
coughing up sputum

Coughing that makes patient dizzy

Loud, rattling breathing

Coughs and bronchitis in the elderly, especially in the winter months

Lips may turn blue

Agg & Alev Conditions

< lying down

> sitting up

> getting the mucus out

NAUSEA/MOTION SICKNESS

Antimonium tartaricum is an important
remedy for the treatment of cholera, since
cholera patients are often nauseated.

General Characteristics

Aversion to touch

Pulse weak and thready

Specific Symptoms

Nausea felt in chest or as a weight on
chest

Intermittent nausea

Retching or vomiting difficult

Nausea and vomiting with a cough

Agg & Alev Conditions

< fever

< worse with   > better with

▶ APIS MELLIFICA

Description

Apis mellifica is made from the whole honeybee.

Dosage

Three or four 30C pellets every 2 to 3 hours until symptoms improve. If there is no improvement after three doses, it is the wrong remedy. Lower doses may also be taken (6C, 6X, 12C, 12X).

Use

BLADDER INFECTION

General Characteristics

Abdomen sensitive to touch

Lack of thirst

Specific Symptoms

Severe pain

Stinging or burning pain

Straining to urinate

Urinating by drops

Strong urge to urinate

May be blood in urine

Involuntary urination from coughing

Scalding pain during urination

Agg & Alev Conditions

< warmth

< night

> cold

CONJUNCTIVITIS

General Characteristics

Busyness

Specific Symptoms

Swelling around the eyes (eyelids may be swollen shut)

Red eyes and eyelids

Gushing hot tears

Stinging, burning eyes

Bloodshot eyes

Agg & Alev Conditions

< heat

> cold applications

HEAT EXHAUSTION

General Characteristics

Lack of thirst

Fainting upon entering a steam bath or sauna

Specific Symptoms

Headache

Red face

Head rolling

Swelling and edema

Agg & Alev Conditions

> heat

INSECT BITES

General Characteristics

Busyness

Specific Symptoms

Bee stings

Burning/stinging

Pink, puffy area

Rapid swelling of part or whole body

Hives

Sensitive and sore skin

Agg & Alev Conditions

< heat

> cold applications

MUMPS

General Characteristics

Lack of thirst

Specific Symptoms

Soft, puffy swelling throughout

Rosy, tender parotid glands

Agg & Alev Conditions

< right side

< heat

> cold

> open air

< worse with   **>** better with

► CHAMOMILLA

Description

Chamomile is a plant from the same family as the common daisy. The whole fresh plant is used to make the homeopathic remedy Chamomilla.

Dosage

Three or four 30C pellets every 2 to 3 hours until symptoms improve. If there is no improvement after three doses, it is the wrong remedy. Lower doses may also be taken (6C, 6X, 12C, 12X).

Use

ASTHMA

General Characteristics

Capriciousness

Tantrums

Children who are irritable, with attacks coming on during or after anger or a tantrum

Desires to be carried

Specific Symptoms

Follows anger

Rattling respiration

Oversensitive to pain

Agg & Alev Conditions

< around 9:00 A.M., 9:00 P.M. to 10:00 P.M.

COLIC

General Characteristics

Capriciousness

Inconsolable

Irritable

Impatient

Specific Symptoms

Comes on after anger

Bloating

Worse during teething

Child wants to be rocked or carried

Green diarrhea that looks like chopped spinach

Agg & Alev Conditions

< warmth

> being carried

EAR INFECTION

General Characteristics

Irritability

Capriciousness

Specific Symptoms

Sensitive, especially to pain

Pale

Child demands to be carried

One cheek red, the other pale

Comes on during teething

Can't bear to be touched or examined

Agg & Alev Conditions

< stooping

< wind

< warm applications

< 9:00 P.M. to midnight

INDIGESTION

General Characteristics

Oversensitive to pain

Specific Symptoms

Comes on after anger or irritation

Belly distended with gas

Cramping

Bitter taste in mouth

Flushed face

Dislikes warm drinks

Stool looks like spinach

Abdominal pain worse with touch and coffee

Agg & Alev Conditions

< after anger

< worse with   > better with

THE PATIENT FILE

Help for a Preschooler's Ear Infection

Like many of the children I see, 4-year-old Sarah had been having recurring ear infections since she was a baby. Her mother came to see me because the antibiotics her doctor prescribed weren't working. On top of that, they caused diarrhea.

Despite the child's obvious discomfort, I explained to her mother that Sarah had to finish all the antibiotics her doctor had prescribed. Otherwise, she might become resistant to certain types of bacteria—and then the antibiotics might not work when Sarah became ill again.

But Sarah clearly needed more than just antibiotics. For immediate comfort, I recommended an even mix of mullein oil and garlic oil—5 drops in each ear, three times a day for a week. This would soothe her discomfort and also help control the infection. I treat both ears because it's not uncommon for bacterial infection to jump from one ear to the other.

I also recommended a homeopathic remedy, 30C of Chamomilla. Chamomilla was indicated because of Sarah's symptoms: She could not bear to be touched or examined, she demanded to be carried or rocked, and she was inconsolable with ear pain. Sarah's symptoms improved after two doses.

Finally, I recommended eliminating dairy foods from Sarah's diet. Generally, children with chronic ear infections are allergic to dairy products. Dairy products contribute to mucus accumulation, and that in turn leads to ear infection. Since Sarah started getting ear infections when her mother switched from breast milk to the bottle, I was pretty sure that eliminating dairy would make a difference. Soy or rice milk and goat's milk are perfectly good substitutes.

I saw Sarah again a week later. The infection and pain were gone.

MENSTRUAL CRAMPS

  General Characteristics

    Extreme irritability

    Demands something, then changes mind as soon as she gets it

    Oversensitive to pain

    Inconsolable

  Specific Symptoms

    Severe menstrual pains that extend to the thighs

    Pain feels as if in labor

  Agg & Alev Conditions

    < at 9:00 A.M. or 9:00 P.M.

    < night

    < after anger

    < coffee

    > being rocked

    > cold applications

TEETHING

  General Characteristics

    Teething accompanied by diarrhea (especially green)

    Inconsolable

    Capriciousness

  Specific Symptoms

    Extreme irritability

    Fussiness

    Terrible tantrums

    Kicking

    Hitting

    Screaming

    Very sensitive to pain

< worse with   > better with

Ear infection

Desires to be carried and rocked

Seizures

Agg & Alev Conditions

< warmth

< pressure

> being carried or rocked

THRUSH

General Characteristics

Irritability

Discontent

Capriciousness

Dislikes attention

Sensitivity to pain

Desires to be carried

Thirst

Specific Symptoms

Complaints about teething

Diarrhea

Fever

Oversensitive to pain

Complaints after anger

Agg & Alev Conditions

< coffee

▶ CHINA OFFICINALIS

Description

The homeopathic remedy China officinalis is made from the plant cinchona, or Peruvian bark. Cinchona is native to the mountain regions of tropical South and Central America and is cultivated in southeast Asia and parts of Africa. Samuel Hahnemann (1755–1843), the founding father of homeopathy, used China officinalis to treat malaria.

Dosage

Three or four 30C pellets every 2 to 3 hours until symptoms improve. If there is no improvement after three doses, it is the wrong remedy. Lower doses may also be taken (6C, 6X, 12C, 12X).

Use

BLEEDING

General Characteristics

Irritability

Sensitivity

Moodiness

Specific Symptoms

Weakness

Faintness

Dim vision

Bleeding with coldness of the body

Gasping or yawning

Profuse bleeding

Agg & Alev Conditions

< touch

< drafts

INDIGESTION

General Characteristics

Irritability

Sensitivity

Touchiness

Specific Symptoms

Comes on after eating fruit

Comes on after abdominal surgery

Belching does not help

Diarrhea worse from fish, fruit, and milk

Bitter taste in mouth

Difficult flatulence

Bloating

Gallbladder pain

Agg & Alev Conditions

< diarrhea

< worse with   > better with

▶ CINNABARIS

Description

Cinnabaris is made from the mineral mercuric sulphide.

Dosage

Three or four 30C pellets every 2 to 3 hours until symptoms improve. If there is no improvement after three doses, it is the wrong remedy. Lower doses may also be taken (6C, 6X, 12C, 12X).

Use

SINUSITIS

General Characteristics

Sensitive to touch

Headache with nosebleed

Specific Symptoms

Pain/pressure in brow, around eyes, and in upper part of nose

Sensation radiates from eyes to side of face

Red eyes

Bloody nose after blowing nose

Stringy mucus running from back of nose to throat, with hawking

Agg & Alev Conditions

< night

< slight touch

> open air

▶ COCCULUS

Description

Cocculus is made from the seeds of the plant *Cocculus indicus*, which is indigenous to Indonesia.

Dosage

Three or four 30C pellets every 2 to 3 hours until symptoms improve. If there is no im-

provement after three doses, it is the wrong remedy. Lower doses may also be taken (6C, 6X, 12C, 12X).

Use

HEADACHE

General Characteristics

Nausea or vomiting brought on by noise

Specific Symptoms

Follows riding in car or boat

Follows strain, overwork, worry, or not sleeping

Agg & Alev Conditions

< noise

> bending head back

INSOMNIA

General Characteristics

Bad effects from grief or anger or from nursing a sick loved one

Specific Symptoms

Insomnia after waking in night

Drowsy but can't sleep

Anxiety dreams

Agg & Alev Conditions

< menstruation

< loss of sleep

NAUSEA/MOTION SICKNESS

General Characteristics

Exhaustion and sickness from anxiety over a loved one

Anxiety

Nervousness

Specific Symptoms

Motion sickness

Dizziness

Metallic taste

Nausea that is worse with motion

Nausea at the mere thought or smell of food

< worse with   > better with

Liver pain and swelling

Worse from anger

Agg & Alev Conditions

< sight, smell, thought of food

< rising

< noise

< fresh air

> lying down

▶ COFFEA CRUDA

Description

Coffea cruda is made from the raw berries of the coffee plant.

Dosage

Three or four 30C pellets every 2 to 3 hours until symptoms improve. If there is no improvement after three doses, it is the wrong remedy. Lower doses may also be taken (6C, 6X, 12C, 12X).

Use

ASTHMA

General Characteristics

Sleeplessness from excitement or joy

Aggravation or nervousness from drinking coffee

Specific Symptoms

Palpitations from excitement

Insomnia with racing thoughts

Agg & Alev Conditions

< excitement, joy

INSOMNIA

General Characteristics

Restlessness

Nervous agitation

Specific Symptoms

Insomnia after excitement or joy

Rush of thoughts

Wide awake at 3:00 A.M. with racing mind

Agitation

Sensitivity to noise, light, and touch

Overstimulation

Hypersensitivity

Agg & Alev Conditions

< noise

< strong odor

< open air

> warmth

▶ COLOCYNTHIS

Description

Colocynthis is made from the fruit of the plant *Citrullus colocynthis*, or bitter apple.

Dosage

Three or four 30C pellets every 2 to 3 hours until symptoms improve. If there is no improvement after three doses, it is the wrong remedy. Lower doses may also be taken (6C, 6X, 12C, 12X).

Use

COLIC

General Characteristics

Restlessness, especially during pains

Oversensitive

Specific Symptoms

Comes on after anger

Severe bloating

Writhing

Restlessness

Pain causes child to bend over

Agg & Alev Conditions

< drinking

< eating (especially fruit)

> doubled up

> bowel movement

> firm pressure to abdomen

< worse with > better with

Chilliness

Shivering

Agg & Alev Conditions

< cold air

< eating

< outdoors

COUGHS

General Characteristics

Sensitivity to noise, odor, light, and music

Specific Symptoms

Dry, teasing cough

Sore larynx and chest

Coughing spells that lead to gagging

Fever

Sour sputum

Shivering

Agg & Alev Conditions

< cold, dry, windy environment

< morning

> hot drinks

DIARRHEA

General Characteristics

Backache

Impatience

Irritability

Specific Symptoms

Comes on after overindulgence (food, alcohol, coffee) or mental exertion

Frequent, small amounts

Urging without bowel movement

Diarrhea from overeating

Sensation that some stool is left in rectum

Agg & Alev Conditions

< anger

< tight clothes

> warm drinks

> bowel movement

EAR INFECTION

General Characteristics

Impatient, ambitious, and driven individuals

Specific Symptoms

Stitching pain

Itching

Increased hearing acuity

Swallowing to relieve itching makes pain worse

Agg & Alev Conditions

< swallowing

HAY FEVER

General Characteristics

Sensitivity

Irritability

Impatience

Specific Symptoms

Sneezing spells

Runny nose indoors/daytime; stopped-up nose outdoors/evening

Symptoms year-round

Nasal discharge from one nostril

Agg & Alev Conditions

< outside

< cold drafts

> indoors

HEADACHE

General Characteristics

Irritable, impatient, ambitious, and driven individuals

Specific Symptoms

Comes on after overindulgence (food, alcohol, coffee) following anger

Hangover

Splitting pain, as if nail driven in

Nausea

Heavy head

Sensitivity to noise, odors, and light

< worse with   > better with

Dizziness

Headache in the sun

Agg & Alev Conditions

< cold

> evening

> rest

INDIGESTION

General Characteristics

Hard-driving individuals

Irritability

Impatience

Specific Symptoms

Comes on after overindulgence (food, alcohol, coffee)

Heartburn

Belching

Bloating

Retching

Needs to loosen belt

Wakes up at 3:00 A.M. from indigestion

Cramping or sharp pains in abdomen

Agg & Alev Conditions

> hot drinks

> vomiting

INFLUENZA

General Characteristics

Irritability

Sensitivity to noise and odor

Specific Symptoms

Cold turns into flu

Chilliness

Nose stuffed up, especially at night

Dislikes being covered even though chilled when not covered

Agg & Alev Conditions

< cold

< open air

> lying down

> warmth

INSOMNIA

General Characteristics

Wants to be the first and best; very competitive

Impatience

Specific Symptoms

Sleepy but can't sleep

Anxious thoughts

Deep sleep just before alarm rings

Follows mental strain

Sensitivity to light, noise, and sound

Irritability in morning

Cannot sleep due to thoughts about work or how to finish task

Sleepiness during the day, worse with eating, sitting, watching TV

Eating too much rich or spicy food or drinking too much alcohol

Agg & Alev Conditions

< after 3:00 A.M.

MENSTRUAL CRAMPS

General Characteristics

Irritability

Impatient, ambitious, competitive, workaholic

Desires any stimulant, such as spicy foods, alcohol, coffee, tobacco

Specific Symptoms

Menstrual pain causes an urge to have a bowel movement

Cramping pains are worse after eating, feeling anger, or drinking alcohol

Agg & Alev Conditions

< anger

< tight clothes

< smoking

< alcohol

< worse with　> better with

> warmth

> warm drinks

NAUSEA/MOTION SICKNESS

General Characteristics

Irritability

Impatience

Specific Symptoms

Comes on after overindulgence (food, alcohol, coffee) or mental exertion

Comes on after anger, irritability, and frustration

Inability to vomit

Retching

Motion sickness

Nausea of pregnancy

Agg & Alev Conditions

< waking

< eating

< anger

< tight clothes

> warm drinks

> after bowel movement

▶ PETROLEUM

Description

Petroleum is made from crude rock oil petroleum.

Dosage

Three or four 30C pellets every 2 to 3 hours until symptoms improve. If there is no improvement after three doses, it is the wrong remedy. Lower doses may also be taken (6C, 6X, 12C, 12X).

Use

HERPES SIMPLEX

General Characteristics

Loses way in well-known streets

Chilliness

Specific Symptoms

Genital herpes

Spreads to anus and thighs

Moist, oozing lesions

Itching

Thick yellow crust on lesions

Agg & Alev Conditions

< open air

> warmth

NAUSEA/MOTION SICKNESS

General Characteristics

Chilliness

Worse from cold temperatures

Specific Symptoms

Motion sickness

Faintness

Paleness

Cold sweat

Excessive salivation

Empty sensation in stomach feels better with eating

Agg & Alev Conditions

< sitting up

< fresh air

< winter

▶ PHOSPHORUS

Description

Phosphorus is made from the mineral phosphorus.

Dosage

Three or four 30C pellets every 2 to 3 hours until symptoms improve. If there is no improvement after three doses, it is the wrong remedy. Lower doses may also be taken (6C, 6X, 12C, 12X).

< worse with   > better with

Use

BLEEDING

General Characteristics

Outgoing

Desires company

Specific Symptoms

Small wounds bleed profusely or easily

Bleeding from blowing the nose

Excessive bleeding from a dental extraction

Profuse uterine bleeding with bright red blood, especially between menstrual periods

Peptic ulcers with bright red blood or coffee-ground color

Agg & Alev Conditions

\> washing face in cold water

\> lying on right side

BURNS

General Characteristics

Anxiety when alone

Thirst for cold drinks

Specific Symptoms

Electrical burns

Agg & Alev Conditions

\< lying on left side

\> eating

COUGHS

General Characteristics

Thirst for ice-cold drinks (including fruit juice)

Desires ice cream

Specific Symptoms

Head cold goes to chest

Dry, tickly, exhausting cough

Chest feels tight or like there is a weight on it

Cough awakens the person

Must sit up because of cough

Every cold goes to the chest

Agg & Alev Conditions

\< lying on left side

\< strong odors

\< talking

\< open air

\< change in temperature

\> lying on right side

\> company

HEADACHE

General Characteristics

Hunger

Acute sense of smell

Specific Symptoms

Pain in forehead

Aches over eyes

Head feels heavy

Desires cold drinks

Face feels flushed and hot

Vertigo

Agg & Alev Conditions

\< fasting

\< cough

\< heat

\< before thunderstorm

\> sleep

\> cold applications

\> open air

INFLUENZA

General Characteristics

Anxiety

Specific Symptoms

May seem well

Possible weakness

Thirst for ice-cold drinks but vomits once drinks become warm in stomach

Laryngitis

Pneumonia on left side of chest

Recurring respiratory infections

Every cold goes to the chest

< worse with　> better with

Tickling cough, worse with change of temperature and better sitting up

Agg & Alev Conditions

< fasting

< spicy and salty foods

> cold drinks

NAUSEA/MOTION SICKNESS

General Characteristics

Outgoing, friendly, desires company

Specific Symptoms

Thirst for cold drinks but vomits once drinks become warm in stomach

Empty/hungry feeling

Nausea of pregnancy

Vomiting bright red blood

Stomach pain relieved by cold drinks

Agg & Alev Conditions

< spicy foods

< warm foods

< fasting

▶ PHYTOLACCA

Description

Phytolacca is made from the root, berries, and leaves of the plant *Phytolacca decandra*, or poke root.

Dosage

Three or four 30C pellets every 2 to 3 hours until symptoms improve. If there is no improvement after three doses, it is the wrong remedy. Lower doses may also be taken (6C, 6X, 12C, 12X).

Use

MUMPS

General Characteristics

Sweatiness

Specific Symptoms

Glands under jaw swollen (hard swelling)

Sensation of tension

Excessive salivation

Breast/ovary/testicle swelling

Painful throat

Pain extends to ears on swallowing

Agg & Alev Conditions

< cold

SORE THROAT

General Characteristics

Cannot swallow anything hot

Specific Symptoms

Body aches

Feverish

Swollen lymph nodes in neck

Throat is dark red, purple, or blue

Pain extends to ears on swallowing

Frequent and painful swallowing

Cold

Pain at base of tongue when tongue extended

Sensation of lump in throat

Agg & Alev Conditions

< warm drinks

> cold drinks

▶ PILOCARPUS JABORANDI

Description

Pilocarpus jaborandi is made from hydrochlorate of pilocarpine.

Dosage

Three or four 30C pellets every 2 to 3 hours until symptoms improve. If there is no improvement after three doses, it is the wrong remedy. Lower doses may also be taken (6C, 6X, 12C, 12X).

< worse with   > better with

Use

MUMPS

General Characteristics

Exhaustion after perspiration

Specific Symptoms

Red face

Breast/ovary/testicle swelling

Excessive salivation alternating with dry
mouth

Thirst

Sweatiness

Agg & Alev Conditions

> after sweating

▶ PODOPHYLLUM

Description

Podophyllum comes from the whole plant
Podophyllum peltatum, or mayapple.

Dosage

Three or four 30C pellets every 2 to 3 hours
until symptoms improve. If there is no improvement after three doses, it is the wrong
remedy. Lower doses may also be taken (6C,
6X, 12C, 12X).

Use

DIARRHEA

General Characteristics

Restlessness

Whininess

Specific Symptoms

Watery, offensive, copious, squirting diarrhea (cramping or painless)

Weakness after bowel movement

Gurgling, rumbling, exhausting diarrhea

Sudden urgency to have a bowel movement

Cramps relieved by holding abdomen and
bending forward

Agg & Alev Conditions

< eating

< early morning

< immediately after drinking

< hot weather

▶ PSORINUM

Description

Psorinum is made from the scabies vesicle,
produced by a mite that infests human skin. It
may be available only by prescription from a
homeopathic practitioner.

Dosage

Three or four 30C pellets every 2 to 3 hours
until symptoms improve. If there is no improvement after three doses, it is the wrong
remedy. Lower doses may also be taken (6C,
6X, 12C, 12X).

Use

ASTHMA

General Characteristics

Chilliness

Individual aggravated by drafts and open
air

Specific Symptoms

Shortness of breath and fatigue

Palpitations when lying on left side

Individual feels better lying on his back
with arms spread out as if crucified

Agg & Alev Conditions

< open air

< cold drinks

< worse with   > better with

▶ PULSATILLA

Description

The homeopathic remedy Pulsatilla is made from the whole plant *Pulsatilla nigricans*, or wind flower.

Dosage

Three or four 30C pellets every 2 to 3 hours until symptoms improve. If there is no improvement after three doses, it is the wrong remedy. Lower doses may also be taken (6C, 6X, 12C, 12X).

Use

ASTHMA

General Characteristics

Sweet/affectionate

Tearful/clingy

Lack of thirst

Specific Symptoms

Phlegm

Sensation of weight on chest

Rattling breath during sleep

Dry cough at night, loosening up in the morning

Shortness of breath

Thick yellow-green nasal discharge

Agg & Alev Conditions

< evening or night

< warm room

> open air

BLADDER INFECTION

General Characteristics

Desires company, attention

Tendency to weep

Warm feeling

THE PATIENT FILE

Help for PMS

A week before her menstrual periods began, 34-year-old Kathy became an emotional mess. One minute she'd be weepy and the next minute irritable. No two periods were the same, but she always suffered from migraines at the end. During her periods, Kathy craved butter, cream, cheese, and ice cream. She drank little water.

All of these symptoms indicated that Kathy was a classic candidate for the homeopathic remedy Pulsatilla. I suggested three or four 30C pellets twice a day just before her period until her symptoms improved, and 50 milligrams a day of vitamin B_6, which also helps relieve premenstrual syndrome. I recommended that Kathy eliminate caffeinated beverages and alcohol from her diet, and that she eat four or five small protein meals a day to regulate her blood sugar and balance her mood.

One month later, she said that she had been less emotional around her menstrual period—and less irritable around her boyfriend. She didn't even get a migraine when her period ended. I told her to stop taking the homeopathic remedy but continue taking the supplements.

Specific Symptoms

Urge to urinate when lying on back

Stress incontinence (when coughing, laughing, running)

Urine in dribbles or copious amounts

Spasmodic pain

< worse with > better with

Agg & Alev Conditions

< warmth

< after urination

< pregnancy

< coughing

> cool

CHICKENPOX

General Characteristics

Tendency to weep

Clinginess

Lack of thirst

Specific Symptoms

Nausea

Cough

Enlarged lymph nodes

Itching worse when overheated

Agg & Alev Conditions

< evening

< heat

< change in weather

> cold applications

> motion

> open air

COLDS

General Characteristics

Lack of thirst

Tendency to weep

Desires attention/sympathy

Desires open air

Specific Symptoms

Thick, creamy, yellow nasal discharge

Nose stopped up at night and when indoors; nose runny when outdoors

Chapped lips

Cannot smell because nose is stopped up

Spasmodic coughing leads to gagging

Cough worse with exertion, lying down, at night

Agg & Alev Conditions

> motion

> open air

CONJUNCTIVITIS

General Characteristics

Changeable emotions

Cries easily

Specific Symptoms

Thick, watery, yellow-green discharge from eyes

Itching and burning of eyes and eyelids, especially in babies

Agg & Alev Conditions

< evening

< warm room

> open air

> cold applications

COUGHS

General Characteristics

Tendency to weep

Lack of thirst

Specific Symptoms

Dry in evening and loose in morning

Coughing spells lead to gagging

Thick yellow sputum

Sensation of weight on chest

Rattling breath during sleep

Must be propped up to sleep because of cough

Agg & Alev Conditions

< warm room

> sitting up

> open air

EAR INFECTION

General Characteristics

Tendency to weep

Lack of thirst

Desire for attention

< worse with   > better with

Specific Symptoms

Red, swollen outer ear

Severe, throbbing pain in inner ear, outer ear, or both

Sensation of stopped-up ear

Diminished hearing

Discharges from the ears (also called glue ears)

Agg & Alev Conditions

< heat

< evening

> open air

HEADACHE

General Characteristics

Tendency to weep

Desire for company

Specific Symptoms

Follows rich foods, fright, or exposure to sun

Nausea/vomiting

Pain changes location

Throbbing pain

Occurs at the last hour of menstrual flow

Flushes of heat to the face

Agg & Alev Conditions

< sun

< exertion

> firm pressure

> slow walking

> open air

> cold applications

INDIGESTION

General Characteristics

Irritability

Changeable symptoms

Weepy, moody

Specific Symptoms

Comes on after eating rich foods

Dry mouth

Bad taste in mouth

Lack of thirst

Need to loosen belt

Thick white or yellow coating on tongue

Craves fatty foods that individual cannot digest

Gurgling or rumbling abdomen at night

Agg & Alev Conditions

< night

< warm drinks

> cold drinks

INSOMNIA

General Characteristics

Hot feet

Desires attention

Lack of thirst

Specific Symptoms

Frequent waking

Sleepy but can't sleep

Recurring thoughts

Sensitive to noise

Sleep disturbed by a particular song running through individual's mind

Sleeps on abdomen or back with arms raised over head

Agg & Alev Conditions

< heat

< rich foods

< before midnight

> open air

MEASLES AND RUBELLA

Pulsatilla is recommended in the later stages of measles or rubella, when the child has a high fever.

General Characteristics

Desires company, attention

Whininess

Tendency to weep

Lack of thirst

< worse with   > better with

Specific Symptoms

Cough that is dry at night and loose in day

Thick yellow nasal discharge

Watery eyes

Rash becomes large pustules

Agg & Alev Conditions

< heat

< dusk

> cool air

> day

MENSTRUAL CRAMPS

General Characteristics

Very changeable moods

One minute weepy, the next minute irritable

Shyness or bashfulness

Craves sweets, cream, butter, cheese

Specific Symptoms

No two periods are the same

Menstrual periods are irregular

Pain with the menstrual cycle

The pain causes the person to cry

Headaches occur at the end of the menstrual flow

Menstrual pain since puberty

Agg & Alev Conditions

< sun

< evening

< before or during menstruation

MUMPS

General Characteristics

Tendency to weep

Whininess

Needs others near when sick

Lack of thirst

Specific Symptoms

Long-lasting illness

Painful, swollen parotid glands

Breast/ovary/testicle swelling

Agg & Alev Conditions

< warmth

< lying down

< night

> open air

> cold applications

PREMENSTRUAL SYNDROME

General Characteristics

Changeable moods

Alternately weepy, irritable

Shyness, bashfulness

Craves sweets, cream, butter, cheese

Faints in warm or stuffy rooms

Specific Symptoms

Irregular menstrual periods

Painful menstruation

Changeable menstrual flow

Headache at the end of menstrual flow

Agg & Alev Conditions

< sun

< evening

< fatty or rich foods

< before or during menstruation

SINUSITIS

General Characteristics

Irritability

Tendency to weep

Lack of thirst

Specific Symptoms

Thick yellow-green nasal discharge

Stuffy nose with a loss of smell

Agg & Alev Conditions

< night

< warm room

< standing

< stooping

< raising eyes

> morning

< worse with   > better with

> pressure

> open air

STY

General Characteristics

Changeable moods

Tendency to weep

Clinginess

Specific Symptoms

Yellow-green pus

Dry eyes

Feels as if foreign body is in eyes

Tears

Feels like rubbing eyes

Thick, watery, yellow discharge

May experience pain and itching of the eyes

Agg & Alev Conditions

< warmth

> open air

> cold applications

VAGINITIS

General Characteristics

Lack of thirst

Changeable emotions

Tendency to weep

Specific Symptoms

Milky, creamy, or yellow discharge

May occur during pregnancy

May occur during puberty

Changeable menstrual flow

Itching and burning (scratching makes the itching and inflammation worse)

Agg & Alev Conditions

< heat

< lying down

> cool

VARICOSE VEINS

General Characteristics

Sweet, affectionate

Weepy, clingy

Changeable moods

Specific Symptoms

Restlessness

Redness and swelling

Tearing, stinging, sharp, intense pain

Pain changes location

Agg & Alev Conditions

< during pregnancy

> cold

▶ PYROGENIUM

Description

Pyrogenium is made from decomposed lean beef. It may be available only by prescription from a homeopathic practitioner.

Dosage

Three or four 30C pellets every 2 to 3 hours until symptoms improve. If there is no improvement after three doses, it is the wrong remedy. Lower doses may also be taken (6C, 6X, 12C, 12X).

Use

INFLUENZA

General Characteristics

Flaring nostrils

Talkative

Specific Symptoms

Looks sick

Bone pain

Restlessness

Hurts to move and bed feels hard

Offensive-smelling secretions

Very shiny red tongue

Rapid fever

< worse with   > better with

Chills start between shoulder blades

Thirst

Aching throughout whole body

Agg & Alev Conditions

> heat

> hot bath

> pressure

SINUSITIS

General Characteristics

Restlessness during fever

Specific Symptoms

Foul nasal discharge

Fever

Agitation

Aching throughout body

Throbbing headache is better with pressure

Agg & Alev Conditions

< cold, dampness

> heat

> pressure

▶ RANUNCULUS BULBOSUS

Description

Ranunculus bulbosus comes from the plant of the same name, which is commonly known as buttercup.

Dosage

Three or four 30C pellets every 2 to 3 hours until symptoms improve. If there is no improvement after three doses, it is the wrong remedy. Lower doses may also be taken (6C, 6X, 12C, 12X).

Use

SHINGLES

General Characteristics

Irritability

Touchiness

Specific Symptoms

Lesions on chest or back

Intercostal neuralgia, especially on the lower left side of the chest

Severe pain

Bluish lesions with blood-stained fluid

Agg & Alev Conditions

< deep breath

< touch

< motion

< lying on affected side

> being still

▶ RHUS TOXICODENDRON

Description

The homeopathic remedy Rhus toxicodendron comes from the shrub of the same name, which is commonly known as poison oak. The remedy is made from the leaves of the plant.

Dosage

Three or four 30C pellets every 2 to 3 hours until symptoms improve. If there is no improvement after three doses, it is the wrong remedy. Lower doses may also be taken (6C, 6X, 12C, 12X).

Use

CHICKENPOX

General Characteristics

Restlessness

Chilliness

Tip of tongue red

Specific Symptoms

Extreme itchiness made worse by scratching

Cannot find a comfortable position

Rash becomes large pustules

< worse with   > better with

respiratory ailments such as chronic cough, shortness of breath, and asthma as well as hoarseness, painful diarrhea, fatigue, and skin problems.

Liver/Gallbladder. The Heart might govern circulation, and the Spleen might maintain the blood in your blood vessels, but the Liver regulates the volume of blood that circulates within you. It also makes sure that qi flows smoothly throughout the body and nourishes your eyes and all of the tendons that connect your muscles to your bones. The Liver is also involved in the expression of anger. The Gallbladder performs similar functions, in addition to its unique role of storing bile for digestion.

As you might expect, a qi imbalance in this system can cause tendon problems, constriction in the upper abdomen, and vision-related disorders. But because this energy meridian encircles the genitals, it also affects menstruation and the health of the penis and vagina. Anxiety or depression also may result from an imbalance here.

Kidney/Bladder. Water metabolism is only one of the Kidney system's responsibilities, according to TCM theory. These organs also regulate growth, produce bone marrow, receive qi from the Lungs, serve as the foundation of yin and yang for the whole body, and store your "essence," your genetic heritage. Last, whenever you feel afraid of something, the Kidney system is in some way implicated.

While an imbalance in the Triple Burner may cause ear problems, the kidneys actually rule over your aural health. The Bladder, meanwhile, does what you would expect it to do—store and dispense with urine. Urinary difficulties can arise when qi within this system is disturbed. You also might experience pain in your knees or lower back, bone disorders, and developmental problems, including premature aging.

The Test of Time

When speaking of Traditional Chinese Medicine, have you ever stopped to wonder just how long Asian healers have been following the tradition?

In the early 1970s, in China's Hunan Province, archaeologists discovered a tomb built sometime between 206 B.C. and A.D. 220. Among the artifacts found inside was a medical book, entitled *Wu Shi Er Fang*, which translates as "Formulas for the Treatment of 52 Diseases."

Believed to have been written between 403 B.C. and 221 B.C., the tome is the oldest record of Chinese medicine ever discovered.

THE FIVE ELEMENTAL ENERGIES

The Five Elemental Energies—Fire, Earth, Metal, Water, Wood—are fundamental forces of nature whose constant transformations and interactions make the world go around. All living things contain the Five Elemental Energies in various proportions. These Energies transform, manifest, and maintain their own natural equilibrium while remaining in dynamic flux. The Chinese Medicine practitioner administers herbs that have governing Elemental Energies. These governing Energies give herbs specific affinities for ailing organs and their associated energy channel. By using the Five Elemental Energies, the TCM practitioner can balance and harmonize the vital energies involved in regulating human health.

There are Creative cycles and Control cycles that govern the relationships among the Five Elemental Energies. The Creative cycle represents the way in which the different Elements nourish

Energy	Flavor	Color	Yin	Yang
Fire	Bitter	Red	Heart	Small Intestine
Earth	Sweet	Yellow	Spleen/Pancreas	Stomach
Metal	Pungent	White	Lungs	Large Intestine
Water	Salty	Black	Kidneys	Bladder
Wood	Sour	Green	Liver	Gallbladder
Fire II	Bitter	Red	Pericardium	Triple Burner

and support each other. The Control cycle represents the way in which the different Elements hold each other in check, like the spokes in a wheel. In the Creative cycle, Wood generates Fire, Fire generates Earth, Earth generates Metal, Metal generates Water, and Water generates Wood. In the Control cycle, Metal holds Wood in check, Wood holds Earth in check, Earth holds Water in check, Water holds Fire in check, and Fire holds Metal in check.

Each pair of the yin and yang organs is also governed by one of the Five Elemental Energies. For example, the Heart (yin) and the Small Intestine (yang) are ruled by Fire energy. The Kidney (yin) and Urinary Bladder (yang) are ruled by Water energy. If, for example, the Water energy of the Kidney is deficient, it loses control of the Fire energy of the Heart due to imbalances in the Control cycle (Water holds Fire in check). In this case, the Fire energy of the Heart can flare up and burn out of control, giving rise to symptoms such as insomnia, heart palpitations, tongue ulcers, restlessness, and a rapid pulse. In conventional medicine, these symptoms will be treated as a heart problem; but in TCM, the root cause of the problem is deficient Kidney energy. The TCM practitioner will treat this condition by prescribing herbs to nourish and increase the Water energy of the Kidney.

Another manifestation of the Five Elemental Energies in nature are the five flavors. The Five Flavors are one of the ways by which the therapeutic properties of medicinal herbs are identified. For example, sweet herbs have the property of Earth energy and can therefore be used for ailments of the Stomach and Spleen/Pancreas. Most medicinal herbs contain more than one energy and flavor and can be used to treat more than one organ system. When combined in complex formulas, the Elemental Energies of the herbs mix and metabolize in complex ways in the human body. This is why extensive clinical experience is so important in prescribing Chinese herbal medicines.

THE SIX CLIMATIC PATHOGENS

In conventional medicine, viruses and bacteria are the primary culprits in causing disease. In Traditional Chinese Medicine, there are six primary pathogens. These are: Wind, Cold, Fire, Summer-Heat, Dampness, and Dryness. These are all natural phenomena and are not in themselves harmful. If, however, a person with a yin and yang imbalance is exposed to extremes of these climatic pathogens, he can develop symptoms of disease.

Wind. Wind is a natural climatic phenomenon. When we are too hot, wind can cool our bodies. According to TCM, Wind can be a good or a bad influence on our health, depending on the circumstance. It is considered to be yang in nature and tends to injure the yin and blood of the body. Wind, when it attacks the body, tends to move upward and stay high. It often attacks the upper region of the body, causing headaches or coldlike symptoms. Wind also can move fast and is constantly changing, causing symptoms to move from one place to another. For example, rheumatism characterized by pain that moves from one part of the body to another is caused by Wind.

Cold. Cold is the dominant climate in the winter months. Cold can attack the body superficially or penetrate more deeply into the body. Cold is considered yin in nature and damages the yang of the body. Common symptoms when Cold attacks the superficial region of the body include fever without perspiration, a headache with a stiff neck, pain in the bones, or a severe fixed pain with difficulty moving the affected part. Cold can also attack deeper regions of the body, causing symptoms such as fatigue, a pale complexion, cold sensations in the limbs that are relieved by applications of heat, watery stool or diarrhea in the morning, and abdominal pain and swelling of the extremities. Other symptoms of Cold invasion include chilliness, numbness of the feet and arms, slow and feeble breathing, spasmodic pain, and purple-colored skin.

Summer-Heat. Heat is considered yang in nature and injures the yin and the fluids of the body. Summer-Heat invasion is a phenomenon that occurs only in the summer months. Common symptoms associated with Summer-Heat invasion of the body are aversion to heat, sweating, headache, dry lips, thirst, and scanty, dark urine. Summer-Heat is harmful because the body loses moisture. In serious cases, Summer-Heat can invade the Heart and can result in symptoms such as delirium and unconsciousness.

Dampness. An individual who walks in the rain or lives in a damp climate, sleeps on damp ground, or swims a lot can be an easy target for an invasion of Dampness. Dampness is considered yin in nature and damages the yang aspects of the body. Symptoms associated with Dampness include arthritis, rheumatism, headaches, swelling of the lower limbs, frequent and difficult urination, vaginal discharge between periods, feelings of heaviness or stuffiness, and thirst without the desire to drink.

Dryness. Dryness is the main climate in autumn. It is yang in nature and damages the yin and the fluid of the body. Dryness can easily harm the lungs, causing a dry cough, a sore throat with dryness, dry skin, dry nasal passages, thirst, scanty urine, and constipation. An internal Dryness can also be caused by excessive consumption of alcohol and hot spices, or when Fire damages the fluids of the body.

Fire. Fire is needed by the body to maintain normal body temperature. Fire is yang in nature and damages the yin and the fluid of the body. Too much anger, exposure to extremely high temperatures, eating spicy foods, and the use of alcohol and cigarettes can generate Fire in the

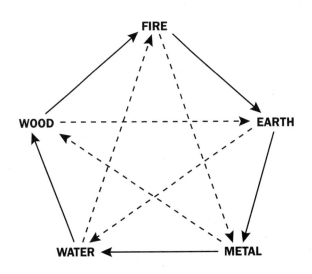

body. Common symptoms of Fire include cracked lips, extreme thirst, insomnia, backache, profuse perspiration, cough, and asthma. In severe cases, too much Fire can cause a high fever, migraine headaches, vomiting, diarrhea, and bleeding.

WHY YOU GET SICK

In TCM theory, disease occurs for either internal or external reasons. An internal cause is some sort of glitch or dysfunction in one or more of the organ systems; an external cause is an intrusion by a pathogen. Whatever the cause, the resulting condition is either excessive or deficient in nature, or perhaps a little of both. Given the seesaw relationship between yin and yang, an excess of one element typically results in a deficiency of another.

Traditional Chinese practitioners recognize that the six climatic pathogens detailed above interact with one another and can each be caused by external forces or internal turbulence.

You can have a heat-related syndrome, for example, because of an external element, such as overexposure to the sun, or because of a deficiency of yin, given that yin tends to be cooling in nature. Similarly, you might have a dampness-related syndrome if you got caught in a rainstorm without an umbrella on a chilly fall day, or because you have a problem with your spleen, which transforms and transports water through the body.

In diagnosing health problems, Traditional Chinese physicians rise to a threefold challenge. They determine if the ailment is deficient or excessive in nature, they figure out which organ systems are affected, and they learn which pathogens might be present.

The distinctions are vital, for they determine the appropriate treatment. It's not enough to

What Is a Chinese Patent Formula?

The Traditional term for the patent medicines covered in this section is *Zhong Cheng Yao*. *Zhong* means "Chinese"; *Cheng* means "prepared," or ready to be taken; *Yao* means "medicine." The Chinese produce and use them because they are *Yan Bian Lian*: effective, convenient, and economical.

Chinese patent medicines, whose history spans more than 2,000 years, are made with standard formulas and standard methods of production. In the 1950s, the Chinese government set national standards for these formulas after holding a series of meetings with manufacturers in different regions of the country and selecting the best method of production. In 1977, the government produced an authoritative resource, titled *The Pharmacopoeia of the People's Republic of China*, which covered 270 standardized patent medicines. All of the patent formulas included in this book are standardized by the Chinese government.

Today, Chinese patent formulas are manufactured not only in China but also in the United States and other countries. All formulas manufactured in China are regulated by the FDA, although some contain synthetic drugs, colorings, and other additives that may be unhealthy. Therefore, it's best to purchase Chinese patent formulas that are made in the United States whenever possible. Formulas purchased from a Chinese grocery store are likely to be imported from China, but because of the ban on synthetic drugs, most health food stores carry only formulas manufactured in the United States.

know only that someone is coughing. A cough might be caused by rebellious qi in the lungs, a deficiency of yin, or excess dampness. Each cause demands an entirely different herbal formula.

HOW FORMULAS ACHIEVE BALANCE IN THE BODY

TCM practitioners designed herbal formulas with several aims in mind. The formulas buck up a deficiency or tone down an excess, they restore the yin-yang balance to the out-of-kilter organ system, and they remove pathogens and toxins.

If you're coughing up clear or white sputum, you have wind-cold syndrome and require a certain treatment formula. If you're coughing up thick, yellow sputum, you have wind-heat syndrome and need something entirely different. Whatever the specific symptoms, chances are that TCM has a specific formula.

Notice the use of the word *formula*. You can purchase many herbs individually today at health food stores, drug stores, even supermarkets. Rarely, however, will a TCM practitioner prescribe an individual herb. Most Traditional Chinese treatments combine at least two and as many as dozens of herbs along with animal products into special, specific formulas.

Why? Because the body's intricate and delicate balance between yin and yang rarely hinges on a single factor. One disruption produces many related disruptions. Each facet must be addressed. Each must be quelled, satisfied, restored, redressed, rebalanced. What's more, prescribing a single herb might create yet another imbalance somewhere in the body.

Many people take ginseng, a widely available supplement, to increase their energy levels. Few

Animal Products in Chinese Formulas

We've all read stories or watched television programs about elephants, rhinoceroses, tigers, and other majestic beasts being threatened with extinction because of poachers, who kill for animal parts that are highly desired among practitioners of Traditional Chinese Medicine.

Elephant tusk, rhino horn, tiger bone, and other exotic animal parts command a high price, particularly in China and specifically because of their therapeutic value in Traditional Chinese Medicine.

A number of Chinese formulas contain animal products. Rhinoceros horn is said to help with blood heat. Gallstones from oxen are said to be useful in treating heat and spasms. Tiger bones are said to be useful against pain and spasms. A yang-boosting tonic might contain deer antler, gecko lizard, the male genitalia of various animals, or even human placenta.

If you object to the inclusion of animal products on humane or vegetarian grounds, make sure you read the labels on Traditional Chinese formulas before you purchase or ingest them, or consult with a practitioner. A knowledgeable traditional Chinese healer can alert you to the presence of animal products in any treatment and can propose a substitute formula.

classically trained Chinese practitioners would recommend taking only this herb because exclusive or unlimited use of the yang-leaning ginseng can create a yin deficiency. Similarly, ma huang (ephedra) is another popular Asian supplement that a lot of people turn to as a weight-loss aid. However, its energetic properties can upset your body's balances and lead to high blood pressure, restlessness, tremors, and insomnia.

IMPORTANT SAFETY PRECAUTIONS

In the dosages indicated in this book, prescribed by TCM practitioners and supplied in supplements readily available at health food stores and Chinese grocery stores and pharmacies, Chinese treatments are not toxic. (See "Treating Yourself vs. Consulting a TCM Doctor.") That fact, however, does not mean that you can take TCM treatments lightly. Always keep in mind the following safety concerns.

Dosages. It is important to note that, except where specifically noted, the amounts recommended in this book are for adults. Children must take reduced dosages adjusted for their smaller size. If the label does not suggest a child-sized amount, talk to a TCM practitioner. Note that Chinese patent formulas are not measured in specific sizes, weights, or measurements.

Drug interactions. Traditional Chinese formulas were devised long before the advent of the pharmaceutical industry, and little is known about possible interactions between prescription medications and herbs. Tell your regular physician about any herbal formulas you might want to take. Likewise, tell your TCM practitioner about any pharmaceuticals a doctor has prescribed for you.

Frequency. Don't take any formula indefinitely. If your health problem worsens or does not improve within a few days, see a health care provider.

Pregnancy. No Chinese formula should be taken during pregnancy unless it clearly states that it is specific for pregnancy. Expectant mothers should take Chinese formulas only under the watchful supervision of an experienced

Treating Yourself vs. Consulting a TCM Doctor

Most of the herbal formulas mentioned in this section of the book are readily available from groceries and pharmacies in Chinese neighborhoods in any large city. You may also obtain them from TCM-oriented doctors, acupuncturists, and pharmacists, and health food stores are carrying them in growing numbers. (See "What Is a Chinese Patent Formula?" on page 466.)

Your best bet, though, is to consult first with a skilled, trained Traditional Chinese healer.

The formulas cited herein are the most commonly used and least toxic of all TCM treatments. Despite their potency, they are quite safe. Nevertheless, they will effect changes in your body. They will treat illness, adjust the flow of your qi, and influence how your organ systems function and interact with one another. For these reasons, before you select and take any particular formula, you must ensure that your symptoms match those described as closely as possible.

Formulas with the same name may differ from manufacturer to manufacturer, and the packaging may not contain a complete list of ingredients. Whenever you have any doubt or uncertainty, check with a Traditional Chinese practitioner.

health care practitioner. Chinese herbs, as well as many other drugs, can be teratogenic, causing malformation in the fetus, and are therefore not allowed during pregnancy.

Side effects. Certain herbs will induce noticeable side effects in sensitive people. Rhubarb rhizome, to name one, might cause diarrhea, while ephedra might make you feel nervous or

Glossary of Chinese Medical Terms

Clears means to move excess Heat out of the body, as by opening the channels of the Large Intestine.

Cools means to increase the yin aspect of the body, thus reducing the effects of too much Heat.

Detoxifies means to remove the poisonous effects of too much Fire in the body.

Discharges means to get rid of excess Fire in the Liver. Common symptoms of Liver Fire include headache, dizziness, ringing in the ears, deafness, jumpiness, red complexion, burning pain in the rib region, vomiting of blood, dark urine, and dry stool.

Dispels means to move excess Wind and Heat from the thoracic area.

Eliminates means to get rid of an excess, such as Dampness, that is causing a health condition.

Expels means to direct out of the body.

Harmonizes means to balance yin and yang in the body, which often increases function; for example, harmonizing the Stomach aids digestion.

Invasion means penetrating the defenses of the body; for example, one may be taken over by Wind and Cold.

Jing means "essence." The Kidney stores jing, which determines one's vitality, resistance to disease, and longevity. One is born with a congenital jing, which influences individual constitution and development.

Lower Burner means the pelvic cavity.

Meridians are channels or pathways through which qi flows in the body.

Middle Burner means the abdominal cavity.

Moistens means to increase the moisture or yin of the body, thus decreasing Dryness.

Moves means to move stagnant qi or blood.

Quells means to stop Fire from moving upward in the body. Common symptoms of ascending Fire include dizziness and high blood pressure.

Raises means to lift up the yang qi, or increase the yang energy in the body.

Regulates means to bring the qi of the organs in the Middle Burner, or abdomen, into balance.

Resolves means to eliminate Dampness and Heat in the Gallbladder.

Sedates means to calm down, such as calming the Fire in the Liver.

Shen means "spirit" and encompasses emotions as well as mental functions such as memory and mental activity. Treatments are often focused on calming the spirit.

Stagnation refers to an obstruction in the free and smooth flow of qi or blood through the body. Factors that can cause qi stagnation include stress, irregular eating, and traumatic injuries; common symptoms include dull pain, swelling, swollen breasts, abdominal distention and pain, irritable bowels, dysmenorrhea, and metrorrhagia. Signs of stagnant blood include a stabbing pain that is fixed in one area, frequent bleeding, bleeding with dark purple clots, and dark purple tongue with red spots.

Tonifies means to build up and strengthen one's qi, blood, and wei (defensive energies).

Toxic means bad or poisonous to the body.

Triple Burner is the area around the pericardium (the lining around the heart). What the Triple Burner fully represents continues to be the subject of great debate. In practice, the Triple Burner is most often seen as having three functions: to transport original qi from the Kidney to the five yin and yang organs; to assure the free flow of water and body fluids through the body; and to represent the health and pathology of three divisions of the body—the Upper, the Middle, and the Lower Burners.

Upper Burner is the thoracic cavity.

prevent you from falling asleep. If a new concern arises after you begin to take a TCM treatment, stop taking the formula and consult a trained pracitioner.

Switching medications. Chinese medicines should not be considered to be a replacement for any other medication you are currently taking. Before switching to Chinese medicine or any other kind of medicine, or before adding it to your current medical regimen, be sure to consult a health care practitioner and be monitored during the transition.

Chinese Research Today

There is very little research done on Chinese medicines today. Chinese herbs have the same problem as Western herbs and supplements: No one wants to invest money in a natural product because natural products cannot be patented. By patenting a product, as in drugs, a manufacturer can make a lot of money.

Most of the research that is done today is on one Chinese herb at a time for a particular disease. This research is mainly done by drug manufacturers looking to find the next magic bullet. Practitioners in Chinese medicine are unable to use these studies because combination herbs are given to patients according to their symptoms. Rarely is just one herb given for a particular illness.

Initial U.S. attempts at clinical research into Chinese medicines have suffered from a lack of adequate funding, insufficient focus on a testable hypothesis, methodological flaws, and reporting bias. At least two studies funded by the National Institutes of Health Office of Alternative Medicine involved Chinese herb prescribing. Both studies were given only $30,000 each, while drugs are regularly granted millions of dollars. Neither of these studies is complete because of the methodological problems discussed below.

The reason that Chinese medicine is widely practiced in China today is mainly financial. It was not until the Chinese revolution in 1949, which caused many Western physicians to leave China, that Traditional Chinese Medicine became valued again. Prior to the revolution, there was a period in China when modern medicine was becoming more accepted and Traditional Medicine was not as valued. With Western physicians leaving, China was faced with a medical crisis. The average Chinese family did not have much money and so looked to Traditional Medicine to treat many diseases.

Much of the research done today in China is limited to publication in Chinese-language journals because the budget for this research comes from the Chinese government. A few translations of varying quality and with varying amounts of original material included are printed in journals and newsletters published in the United States and England, but little attention is paid to the methodology that has been employed.

Chinese researchers do not use the standard research method of modern medicine, the placebo-controlled double-blind study, as a testing tool. Because of this, there is a philosophical divide between Chinese and Western researchers and physicians. Chinese doctors do not diagnose an illness the same way as Western physicians. Chinese medicine uses the pulse-and-tongue diagnosis method. A person can have more heat signs, a deficient qi, or more cold signs, and he is treated accordingly. Western medicine generally recommends anti-inflammatory and pain medications for arthritis. Chinese doctors prefer to use complex herbal de-

HOW TO USE THE CHINESE MEDICINES SECTION OF THIS BOOK

This section covers 79 Chinese patent formulas available in the United States to treat health conditions. Each entry includes the English name by which the formula is most commonly known; the symptoms that the formula treats; the ingredients of the formula, including their Chinese, English, and Latin names; the recommended dosage; and cautions. Also included is important

coctions or pills and tend to adjust the formulas to the needs of the individual patient, especially since patients with the same disease can be treated many different ways. Assigning one treatment over another rather than letting the patient choose, or having the practitioner select therapies according to what seems most appropriate, is inconsistent with Chinese health care practices. One rarely sees a placebo-controlled study involving a life-threatening ailment. In China, placebo-controlled studies tend to involve short-term risk reduction studies that address such problems as lowering cholesterol. Double-blind studies usually compare two agents that are presumed effective, such as an herb and a synthetic drug, rather than an herb and a placebo. The Chinese feel that giving a placebo to a suffering patient is unethical.

The few randomized, controlled, blinded studies conducted in China usually involve isolated active constituents of plants that can be blinded easily with standard drugs or a placebo. The researchers usually select diseases for study according to current Western medical categories and priorities. While this research yields results that can be appreciated worldwide, it doesn't reflect much on what practitioners of Traditional Chinese Medicine do. Therefore, this research may be of interest only to drug companies seeking new patentable drugs.

Those in the United States and Europe who are involved with translating and publishing Chinese journal reports are generally interested in addressing the needs of the practitioners of TCM, where the focus is on making a diagnosis according to the Oriental categories of syndromes and figuring out which herbs to prescribe. As a result, the carefully controlled studies are usually not the ones translated into English. The drug companies seeking new products will not publicize the translated work that they sponsor because their investment goes toward in-house patented-product development.

Given the lack of randomized, blinded, controlled trials in English journals, the determined level of success of Chinese medical interventions is not up to par, according to modern medicine. The debate about research is ongoing. According to Chen Ke-ji, writing in the *Chinese Journal of Integrated Traditional and Western Medicine* in 1995, there are different viewpoints on how to evaluate the progress of TCM. One point of view asserts that there is no need to reassess the effectiveness of TCM because it has been practiced for many centuries—its effectiveness has already been proven. Another view insists on adopting the methods of modern medical science to evaluate the effectiveness of TCM. A third view seeks to integrate the theories and experiences of TCM and modern medicine to design a new program to evaluate the effectiveness of TCM.

information that falls under the following categories.

Symptoms. A symptom set in bold-faced type indicates that it is one of the main symptoms treated by that remedy. **Bold-faced** symptoms are the most important to consider when choosing a Chinese medicine.

Functions. "Functions" explains how each formula acts on the various organ systems of the body (see The Six Organ Systems and Their Intricate Interactions, on page 461). The characteristic functions of the formulas listed are based on diagnostic and historical uses in TCM.

Use. Each patent formula entry includes a use section that lists the diseases and health conditions which the formula may be used to treat. Please note, however, that diagnosing health problems in TCM is an exacting process (see Why You Get Sick, on page 466). For this reason, it is important to consult with a health practitioner trained in TCM.

▶ MING MU DI HUANG WAN

English Name

Bright Eyes Rehmannia Pills

Symptoms

- Dry, itchy, red eyes
- **Excessive tearing**
- **Night blindness**
- **Photophobia**
- Poor vision

Ingredients, in Chinese

Shou Di Huang, Shan Yao, Mu Dan Pi, Fu Ling, Shan Yu Rou, Ze Xie, Gou Qi Zi, Shi Jue Ming, Bai Ji Li

Ingredients, in English (Latin)

Rehmannia Root (Radix Rehmanniae Glutinose Conquitae), Dioscoria Root (Radix Dioscoreae Oppositae), Moutan Root Bark (Cortex Moutan Radicis), Poria Fungus Bark (Cortex Poria Cocos), Asiatic Cornelian Cherry Fruit (Fructus Corni Officinalis), Alisma Rhizome (Rhizoma Alismatis), Lycium Fruit (Fructus Lycii Chinensis), Haliotis Shell (Concha Haliotidis), Tribulis Fruit (Fructus Tribuli Terrestris)

Dosage

10 pills three times a day

Functions

Nourishes Liver and Kidney Yin, sedates Liver Fire, strengthens vision

Cautions

None known

Use

- Night blindness

▶ NAN BAO

English Name

Male's Treasure

Symptoms

- Fatigue
- **Impotence**
- Lower-back pain
- **Lowered sexual drive**
- Poor memory
- **Premature ejaculation**

Ingredients

32 ingredients, including animal parts

Dosage

Two pills twice a day

Functions

Male tonic for deficient Kidney Yang and deficient Spleen Qi and Blood

Cautions

None known

Use

- Impotence

▶ NIU HUANG JIE DU PIAN

English Name

Cow Gallstone Detoxification Tablets

Symptoms

- Dizziness
- Earache
- Fever
- Headache
- **Inflamed sore throat**
- **Mouth and throat dryness**
- Tongue or mouth ulcers
- **Toothache**

Ingredients, in Chinese

Niu Huang, Huang Lian, Bing Pian, Jing Yin Hua, Bo He, Huang Qin, Bai Zhi, Zhi Zi, Da Huang, Chuan Xiong

Ingredients, in English (Latin)

Cattle Gallstone (Calculus Bovis), Coptis Rhizome (Rhizoma Coptidis), Borneol Crystal

(Borneolum), Honeysuckle Flower (Flos Lonicerae Japonicae), Mentha Herb (Herba Menthae), Scutellaria Root (Radix Scutellariae), Angelica Root (Radix Angelicae), Gardenia Fruit (Fructus Gardeniae), Rhubarb Rhizome (Rhizoma Rhei), Ligusticum Rhizome (Rhizoma Ligustici Wallachii)

Dosage

Two pills twice a day

Functions

Clears Heat, detoxifies Fire poison, reduces inflammation

Cautions

Do not use this formula during pregnancy because it can cause miscarriage. Do not use if no heat signs (dry mouth, thirst, fever without chills, or a yellow, coated tongue) are present. May cause diarrhea.

Use

- Fever
- Sore throat
- Toothache

▶ PING CHUAN WAN

English Name

Relieve Dyspnea Pills

Symptoms

- **Shortness of breath that is worse in the evening or with exertion**
- Thin, white sputum

Ingredients, in Chinese

Dang Shen, Ge Jie, Dong Chong Cao, Xing Ren, Chen Pi, Gan Cao, Sang Bai Pi, Bai Qian, Meng Shi, Wu Zhi Mao Tao, Man Hu Tui Zi

Ingredients, in English (Latin)

Codonopsis Root (Radix Codonopsis Pilosulae), Gecko Lizard (Gecko), Chinese Caterpillar Fungus (Cordyceps Sinensis), Apricot Seed (Semen Armeniacae Amarae), Citrus Peel (Pericarpium Citri Reticulatae), Licorice Root (Radix Glycyrrhizae), White Mulberry Bark (Cortex Mori Radicis), Cynanchum Root and Rhizome (Radix et Rhizoma Cynanchi Baiqian), Lapis (Lapis Micae seu Chloriti), (Ficus Simplicissima Lour), (Elaeagnus Glabra Thunb)

Dosage

10 pills three times a day

Functions

Improves shortness of breath, nourishes Lung Yin, stops cough

Cautions

None known

Use

- Bronchitis
- Emphysema

▶ QIAN JIN ZHI DAI WAN

English Name

Woman Stop Vaginal Discharge Pills

Symptoms

- Abdominal distension
- **Fatigue**
- **Lower-back pain**
- Poor appetite
- **Vaginal itching and discharge (white or yellow)**

Ingredients, in Chinese

Dang Gui, Bai Zhu, Xiao Hui Xiang, Yan Hu Suo, Mu Xiang, Xu Duan, Dang Shen, Mu Li, Qing Dai

Ingredients, in English (Latin)

Angelica Dang Gui (Radix Angelicae Sinensis), Atractylodes Rhizome (Rhizoma Atractylodes Macro), Fennel Fruit (Fructus Foeniculi), Corydalis Rhizome (Rhizoma Corydalis), Saussurea

THE PATIENT FILE

Seeing Is Believing

Jim, 59, came to see me because he had several health problems. First, he wanted to lose some weight. Second, he had high cholesterol and high triglycerides (fats stored in the blood). While he had tried prescription drugs to bring his cholesterol level down, nothing had worked. Jim had other problems too. Legally blind for 20 years, he wasn't able to drive and had to use strong eyeglasses and a magnifying glass to read.

Whenever I encounter vision troubles, I detoxify the liver. In Traditional Chinese Medicine, the eyes are a window to the liver, an organ that can become congested by fat, chemicals such as pesticides, and intoxicants including alcohol and tobacco. Cataracts, glaucoma, excessive tearing, nearsightedness, farsightedness, poor night vision, and inflamed, red eyes or dry eyes mirror the condition of the liver.

Because Jim liked to eat soup, I prescribed homemade soups daily for breakfast and lunch. He used fresh herbs that stimulate the liver, such as garlic, ginger, basil, turmeric, bay leaf, cardamom, cumin, fennel, black pepper, and rosemary. I sug-

gested that he add to the soups some cabbage, turnip root, kohlrabi, cauliflower, broccoli, brussels sprouts, artichokes, beets, carrots, and other vegetables that detoxify the liver.

For the evenings, I recommended a dinner menu that included 6 ounces of fish or chicken with a salad, rice, and vegetables. For snacks, I suggested sprouted grain breads, sunflower and pumpkin seeds, and fresh fruits and vegetables. And I suggested that he drink a cup of water with the juice of half a lemon squeezed in. All are good for the liver. Finally, I placed Jim on 500 milligrams of l-carnitine twice a day to lower his triglycerides.

Two months later, Jim came to my office for a follow-up appointment. He had lost 25 pounds. A blood test showed that his cholesterol and triglyceride levels were normal. What's more, he told me that he could see again. A vision test showed that he could read even fine print without his glasses.

Two weeks after that, Jim stopped by my office again, not for a checkup this time, but just to say hello and to show off his driver's license—and his brand-new car.

Root (Radix Saussureae), Dipsacus Root (Radix Dipsaci), Codonopsis Root (Radix Codonopsis Pilosulae), Oyster Shell (Concha Ostreae), Indigo Powder (Indigo Pulverata Levis)

Dosage

10 pills once or twice a day

Functions

Clears Heat and Damp, regulates menstruation, regulates Qi and Blood, stops vaginal discharge

Cautions

None known

Use

• Vaginitis

▶ QI JU DI HUANG WAN

English Name

Lycium Chrysanthemum Rehmannia Pills

Symptoms

• Blurry vision

• **Dizziness**

- **Dry and painful eyes**
- Headache
- Heat in palms
- Insomnia
- **Poor night vision**
- Pressure behind eyes

Ingredients, in Chinese

Shou Di Huang, Shan Yao, Mu Dan Pi, Fu Ling, Shan Yu Rou, Ze Xie, Gou Qi Zi, Ju Hua

Ingredients, in English (Latin)

Rehmannia Root (Radix Rehmanniae Glutinose Conquitae), Dioscoria Root (Radix Dioscoreae Oppositae), Moutan Root Bark (Cortex Moutan Radicis), Poria Fungus Bark (Cortex Poria Cocos), Asiatic Cornelian Cherry Fruit (Fructus Corni Officinalis), Alisma Rhizome (Rhizoma Alismatis), Lycium Fruit (Fructus Lycii Chinensis), Chrysanthemum Flower (Flos Chrysanthemi Morifloii)

Dosage

Eight pills three times a day

Functions

Nourishes Liver and Kidney Yin, nourishes the eyes, strengthens vision

Cautions

None known

Use

- Night blindness

▶ QING FEI YI HUO PIAN

English Name

Clear Lung Eliminate Fire Pills

Symptoms

- Bleeding gums
- **Cough with thick, yellow sputum**
- **Swollen, painful throat**

Ingredients, in Chinese

Huang Qin, Zhi Zi, Da Huang, Qian Hu, Ku Shen, Tian Hua Fen, Jie Geng, Zhi Mu

Ingredients, in English (Latin)

Scutellaria Root (Radix Scutellariae), Gardenia Fruit (Fructus Gardeniae), Rhubarb Rhizome (Rhizoma Rhei), Peucedanum Root (Radix Peucedani), Sophora Root (Radix Sophorae), Trichosanthes Root (Radix Trichosanthis), Platycodon Root (Radix Platycodi), Anemarrhena Rhizome (Rhizoma Anemarrhenae)

Dosage

Four pills twice a day

Functions

Clears Lung Heat, promotes increase in fluids, reduces rising Fire, stops cough

Cautions

Do not use this formula during pregnancy because it may be toxic to the fetus. Do not use if you have signs of cold, such as chills or cold extremities.

Use

- Coughs
- Fever

▶ QING QI HUA TAN WAN

English Name

Clear Lung Energy Eliminate Sputum Pills

Symptoms

- **Coughing so strong it can cause vomiting**
- **Feeling of fullness in chest**
- Fever
- **Strong, loud cough with thick, yellow, sticky sputum**

Ingredients, in Chinese

Ban Xia, Tian Nan Xing, Zhi Shi, Huang Qin, Ju Hong, Gua Lou, Xing Ren, Fu Ling

Underscored page references indicate boxed text.

Inflammation (*continued*)
  joint
    gout, 80
    osteoarthritis, 123–24
    rheumatoid arthritis, 137–38, <u>138</u>
  knee, 122–23
  larynx, 60–61
  lupus, 106
  lymph node, 106–7
  nerve, 121
  periodontium, 130
  sinus, 142, 358–59
  skin
    psoriasis, 134–35
    rosacea, 138
    sunburn, 148–49, 362
  stomach, 78
  throat, 143–44, 359–61
  tongue, 79
  vagina, 153, 364
  vocal cords, 102
Influenza, 96–97, 350–51, <u>403</u>
Infusion, tea, 160
Inosine, 278
Inositol, 278
Insect bites, 97, <u>98</u>, 351
Insomnia, 97–98, <u>111</u>, 352–53
Insulin, 63
Insulin-dependent diabetes, 63–64
Insurance, health, <u>7</u>
Integrated medicine, 8–10, <u>266</u>
Intermittent claudication, 98–99
Iodine, 79–80, 279
Ipecacuanha, 414–15, <u>414</u>
Iris versicolor, 415–16
Iron, <u>15</u>, 37, 99, 279–80
Iron-deficiency anemia, 37, 99–100
Isoleucine, 280

J

Jaundice, 100. *See also* Liver diseases and
    conditions
Jet lag, 100

Jian Bu Hu Qian Wan, 488
Jin Gui Shen Qi Wan, 488
Jing Wan Tong, 489, <u>489</u>
Joint diseases and conditions. *See also* Bone
    diseases and conditions
  gout, 80
  osteoarthritis, 123–24
  pain, 100–101
  rheumatoid arthritis, 137–38, <u>138</u>
Juniper, 204–5

K

Kali bichromicum, 416–17
Kali carbonicum, 417–18
Kali iodatum, 418
Kali muriaticum, 418–19
Kali phosphoricum, 419
Kang Gu Zeng Sheng Pian, 489–90
Kava kava, 205, <u>207</u>
Keloids, 72
Kelp, 205–6
Keratoconjunctivitis sicca, 67
Kidney stones, 101–2
Knee pain, 50
Kreosotum, 419

L

Labels, on homeopathic remedies, <u>320</u>
Labor, difficulties of, 49
Lachesis, 419–21
Lactation, insufficient, 39
Laryngitis, 102. *See also* Sore throat
Laughter, stress management and, <u>18</u>
Lavender, 206
Law of Similars, 7, 319–20
LDL, 90–91
L-dopa, 128
Lead poisoning, 86
Lecithin, 281
Ledum, 421–22
Leg cramps, 102–3

<u>Underscored</u> page references indicate boxed text.

Underscored page references indicate boxed text.

Underscored page references indicate boxed text.

<u>Underscored</u> page references indicate boxed text.

Underscored page references indicate boxed text.

Underscored page references indicate boxed text.